PROSTATE CANCER AND ME...OR YOU, THE TWO STAGES
(Man To Man)

LLOYD MARTIN

ISBN:1468067427
ISBN-13:9781468067422

DEDICATION

To my sons Daniel, Nathan, and Matthew.

CONTENTS

CONTENTS (Cont'd)

ACKNOWLEDGMENTS

Whenever one embarks on a journey to a place that he has never been before, a few items are needed. A map, reliable transportation and good company are just a few of the things required to make your travels a success. A good navigation system isn't bad to have either:

And so, the journey that I embarked upon, though unwillingly and unknowingly, would not have been made possible, least of all enduring without the help of the following individuals:
I would first like to thank my wife Annecia, who was my eyes and ears along this tumultuous road. Her unwavering support kept us on the straight and narrow all throughout this travel and for that I will always be grateful.

Next I would like to thank my two mothers. First, my mother Myrtle Francis who immediately dropped everything to be at my side in every sense of the word and whom I will always love and cherish dearly. Second, my mother-in-law Jennifer Bolvin who has shown her love and support for me in more ways than one.

To my two doctors whose qualities such as persistence, knowledge, skill and compassion took me from diagnosis to treatment. With their help and involvement, my uncertainty coupled with fear of the unknown would soon give way to gratitude and thanks. Thank you Dr. Earl Brown for truly practicing medicine and thank you Dr. Jamison Jaffee for your skill, sense of humor and empathy.

I would also like to thank the nursing staff at Hahnemann University Hospital for their caring nature and dedication to my well being.

Chapter One

Man To Man

Let me begin this story by giving you a picture of myself about two years ago: a 47-year-old man with a beautiful wife, two fine young sons, a nice house, a good job. I have been a hearty man, all things considered, throughout my adult life...strong, too. My build and strength were probably inherited from the hulk of a man I had for a father. I usually went to the gym three times a week, trying to keep to that routine with determination and fervor. Being cognizant of what good health involved and what I should be doing to maintain it, I also regularly scheduled annual checkups with my doctor.

All in all, life was good.

Then I was diagnosed with prostate cancer.

In the course of my treatment, I learned many things- about physical exams, about hospital procedures, about the effects of surgery. I learned that worrisome thoughts and emotions can be just as hard to fight as physical disease. Doctors, if you're fortunate, tell you a little about what they're doing and about what to expect. There's a lot they don't tell you. Mostly, you have to find out on your own

Today, I'm in good shape again and my cancer is gone. But I want to tell you what I found out along the way, and hopefully by the end of my story you will be properly informed. I might even scare you into taking some steps you are avoiding. That's all right. I don't mind scaring you a little into doing what just might be necessary to save your life. You see, often enough it is a scared rabbit who jumps, and most likely jumps out of impending danger or peril. So don't be afraid if you happen to be scared, it might be to your benefit.

I was used to overcoming obstacles from my earliest days. My very first obstacle may have been surviving my birth into this world. I was not expected to live when I was born, or so I was told. Apparently, I hollered like a pig being stuck with a knife, so I was told. At the very least, it seemed I cried more than the normal baby, probably because of an inability to soil my Pampers. Today, I joke that it must have been that early training of my vocal cords that gave me the ability to sing, which I can do fairly well, I must say.

Anyway, I lived, and more obstacles trailed me after that noisy beginning.

I'm not certain if the next one was the need to become a man at the tender age of ten, when I had to protect my little sister and only sib- ling from the brutality of our daddy, a person who did not know how to be a father to us, and who suffered from the disease of *parental deficiency,* having not been "Parented" as a child himself. I can recall standing up to this giant of a man, overcoming my fear of what he could so easily do to me with just a swipe of his powerful hand.

Or maybe the bigger obstacle was a speech impediment that rendered me almost mute. The inability to speak with any kind of fluency had, in fact, paralyzed my soul as a child, and threatened to send me permanently into a world of introversion and silence.

Taking the bull by the horn, I attacked that problem with force and set myself a program of self-improvement—quietly reading to myself, talking out loud to myself, and gradually building up the skills I needed to communicate. Along with skills came a confidence that ended the

fears that were preventing me from acting "normal."
Later on, many people could not believe I was able to speak without any sign of stuttering.

At age thirteen, I faced another obstacle. A bully, a big brute of a fellow about nineteen years old, used to terrorize the students at my middle school during recess. He was like a gorilla on the loose; most people were afraid of him and tried to stay out of his way. His day came, however, when, in the typical fashion of a tyrant, he snatched a prized possession from me. He made a big mistake, though, by turning his back on such a pound-for-pound fearless package as me. I pelted him with rocks and he had to drag himself from the school yard, I pelted him with more rocks, and sent him running.

Let me fast-forward now to the time I became an adult, fell in love, and married for the first time.

My decision to start a family, the aspiration I suppose of most grown men, soon enough came to haunt me in the form of what I call a sailboat marriage. The steering mechanism of that union was wrenched from me by my ex-wife, a woman who actually needed a harness instead of the loving hands and tender affection I tried to offer. I was made to walk the plank, while she, as head pirate, looked on and cheered.

All my manly dignities were stripped from me, and I felt like a thing that had been used and thrown away. I could easily have been the next patient in the local asylum, if I had not checked myself into the "private care" of my essentially positive and determined spirit. I survived that marriage, but the emotional impact it had on me left the deepest wounds and gashes, all of which I had to overcome in time to make my second marriage a success.

So yes, my life has been full of obstacles.

Some were perhaps common to humanity; some were unique to me.

And the details of a few of those personal struggles suggest that I probably should not have come out intact. But certain tenacity served me well and kept me going. I carved out a path for myself that felt good, that worked. And there I was, two years ago, at the mid-life stage of the game, enjoying the satisfying feeling of meandering towards my delta like an accomplished river.

Little did I know that my biggest obstacle was yet to come, my greatest challenge just over the horizon.

Chapter 2

Beginning the Journey: On the Road to a Diagnosis

At the beginning of this book, I stated, "I was diagnosed with prostate cancer." That's a quick and simple statement. In fact, getting to that point was anything but quick and simple. The final word came only after five biopsies with three different urologists, physicians who specialize in dealing with what is called the urogenital system and its diseases.

The road to diagnosis started with my annual physical checkup at my doctor's. I'm a little unusual among male friends and compadres where this is concerned, as many of them think you go to the doctor only when you're sick and when nothing in your traditional arsenal can cure it or is making you feel better. On this particular visit, blood work—that's when the doctor takes a small sample of blood and sends it to be analyzed for possible problems, like high cholesterol and diabetic tendencies—revealed that my Prostate Specific Antigen (PSA) level was high.

The PSA is a protein substance secreted by cells of the prostate, a gland that surrounds the urethra at the base of the bladder. Fluid from the prostate is discharged with sperm. PSA levels indicate when something is wrong with the prostate and have been extensively used to screen for cancer. But there wasn't much cause for alarm right then, as the doctor explained my high reading could have resulted from other factors, like an inflamed or an enlarged gland.

To be on the safe side, however, he recommended that I be checked out by a specialist, one of those urologists.

I had no way of knowing at that point that the curtain was just rising on this play, and that there was a long journey ahead of me. A difficult journey. A journey through the cracks and crevasses of prostate cancer. My first examination and biopsy to determine if I had cancer was soon in the works.

Forget all the medical terms here. Let me tell you man-to-man what is involved in a prostate examination and biopsy, and related tests. Bend down low, fellows, pull up a seat, gather in the amphitheaters. Pour a drink, maybe a stiff one, because you might need a little support as I take you through the experience.

The Prostate Examination

The urologist I saw came into the exam room and greeted me as a new patient. He instructed me to strip from the waist down and lie on the table in a fetal position with my butt slightly hanging off the side. Strapping on a pair of surgical gloves, he readied himself for the examination. To this day, the ominous sound of those gloves as he snapped them onto his hands still rings in my ears. That sound signals the beginning of a most unpleasant cavity excavation. He then proceeded to lubricate my anus with a cold jelly, and rather mechanically announced he'd be conducting "the exam," as he simultaneously inserted his finger into the opening of my alimentary canal—in crude terms, my butt hole.

The feeling that resulted from this action was disgusting and repulsive, to say the least. I cannot imagine that any man would not have a similar reaction; you feel at once invaded, violated, and soiled. Out of some primeval instinct, you want to turn around, grab the chair that's standing next to the exam table, and break this fellow's rib with it. But it was possible to understand now the reason for that announcement, "the exam," because somewhere under a layer of consciousness you remember that the doctor is examining you, not raping you. That was helpful.

After he had made his decision as to the size and feel of the prostate, he announced:

"In a healthy condition, the prostate should be the size of a walnut."

So what, you Frankenstein freak! I found myself thinking.
"Yours, though, is bigger than the average bear."

So that is it, I thought. *I have an enlarged prostate, I can get this fixed and everything should be cool.*

I already had learned that an enlarged prostate makes you pee often, you do not feel emptied when you do pee, and you have to get up often at night, in a rush, to go. All these symptoms I had had. Previously, I just chalked them up to having too much to drink or not exercising enough. So as I lay on that examining table, I was encouraged. Okay, I needed to get back to the gym, I'd been letting myself get a little pudgy lately, and blaming it on being a settled married man with small children. My thoughts were suddenly pierced by another announcement from the doctor.

"The probe," he said.

The probe? Wasn't he just probing around in my universe? What was this about now?

I did not see that probe, and that was fortunate. Had I seen that thing that was about to be shoved inside me, I do believe it would have left a permanent scar on my otherwise clear and sane mind. I certainly *experienced* that probe, however, as a hard implement, cold to the feel and foreign in sensation, was being moved up and around my anal tract.

If the announcement "the probe" hadn't been made, and if the hard examining table and the guy in the white jacket, the little chair, the manila file, if all that had not created an ambience that oriented my mind and senses to the fact that yes, I was in a doctor's office, I would swear that I was being victimized. A burly man with hairy arms, was standing behind me, shoving a metallic instrument up my rear in the name of good health! It is no wonder some other burly men stay away, never get checked, and end up dying from the disease.

Yes, the ambiance of a doctor's place was there, and yet it was tough to keep appreciating this man as a doctor. He was the attacker or the examiner, maybe the bully presenting me with a new obstacle to overcome. I had to fight to bring myself back mentally from the place my mind was taking me. My Jamaican blood was boiling right then for real, and I just wanted to get up and cut this guy or beat him up good, just like I had done with my old enemy in the schoolyard. I worked hard to put some ice water back in my veins.

"Well," the doctor said, "I have not seen anything so far for me to be concerned. Your urine is clear, and that's a good sign, too." At the beginning of our appointment, he had had me pee in a cup for testing purposes.

Okay, I was thinking, *time for me to put my underwear and pants back on, and get the heck out of here.*

Not so fast. The biopsy followed.

You have probably heard the term "biopsy," and perhaps never paid much attention to it. The dictionary definition of biopsy, the removal of a piece of living tissue for the purposes of a diagnostic examination, does not in any way convey the actual experience. Let me give you the actual experience.

The doctor's voice broke the silence. As I think back, I can now appreciate that his voice sounded somewhat different than it had previously. The tone was more serious with intent, as you might sound if you needed to concentrate harder on the task at hand.

"You will hear a snapping sound, like that of a stapler," my doctor/examiner explained, "and you'll feel a corresponding pinch." As I mentioned earlier, I didn't see the tool he was using, but when the process began it reminded me of a shotgun being cranked and rounds squeezed off. As the tool ripped a piece of my prostate out, the pain was instant.

Now, at this stage of the game, I had lost all trust in this fellow. He'd just told me this was going to feel like a pinch. A pinch? Give me a break! A stab, was more like it. The shock to my nerves was tremendous, and what kept me from hollering out, I do not know. Or, in fact I do know.

All my life I was considered to be a tough guy by many, and I had actually lived tough, especially at those times I needed to. Only the toughest of the tough survive in my book. And this was a moment I needed to be tough. I knew I couldn't cry out like a girl and thereby destroy my aura of toughness. I must admit also—forgive me for this confession—that I didn't want to give this sadistic beast (as I was considering him at that point) the satisfaction of realizing he was hurting me. I'm sure the good doctor did not deserve to have me thinking about him in those terms, but it was my way of insulating myself from what I was experiencing.

That was the first round. There was more to come.

On the second round, I had to clench my teeth, or that "click-clang" sound could have been easily followed by "Eh-aaah!," the sound of one now trembling tough guy lying helplessly on the doctor's examining table, clutching desperately onto the sheet coverings. I had to undergo that ordeal twelve times, as twelve little pieces of my intact gland were snipped out.

I imagine some biopsies are harder to tolerate than others, and I also imagine that a biopsy anywhere on the outside of the body would be less traumatizing than one done on the inside, especially on a sensitive gland like the prostate. There was no Novocaine, no dulling of nerves or anything. I thought I knew how a plucked chicken feels, but then it occurred to me that the chicken wouldn't feel anything because it would be dead. I was in a worse situation than a plucked fowl, because I was alive and felt every single pluck, all the way up, up, up in my innards.

At that point, the game should have been over and done with, don't you think? Yes, I thought so, and I couldn't wait to hightail it out of there. Two Scotch on the rocks, I was thinking, that's what it will be when I get out of here, or make that two double shots. Two double shots should help to retrieve my sanity from whatever orbit this experiment or rather experience had sent it into.

So I was relieved when the doctor said, "All right, we're done here, you did good." Then he wiped my rear with some wet, cold stuff and tossed the cleaning material into a bin. I could hear the "clunk" sound as it hit the receptacle, and that sound was significant to me—I think because it signaled some finality. And boy, did I need this ordeal to be finally over.

Patting me on the shoulder and heading for the door, the doctor said, "I'll be right back."

Not such a bad fellow after all, I thought. I had a little chuckle, too, when I remembered that this was the same fellow I wanted to cut or beat up just a few minutes earlier. *Well, anyway, I wouldn't want to do what he does for a living. Can't be so pleasant, sticking your finger inside people and probing around in there. And the smell? How does one stand all those smells? Not me.*

As if the doctor dude had been reading my mind and was aiming to have the last laugh, he reappeared just then and announced, "This is the last thing we have to do."

Okay, so what? I reasoned, *it's the last thing, couldn't be worse than the others, could it?*

Yes. Yes, it could be worse.

The Penile Examination

The next stage in my examination for prostate cancer was the penile insertion, which is a term that I think explains itself. I can appreciate why the word "penile" closely resembles the word "penal," which means punishment. Penile insertion was no joke. It was another walk in proverbial hell, and the devil was this same doctor dude.

Dangling from his right hand now was an implement that looked like a thin black wand, or what jockeys use in the sport of kings to get the thoroughbreds moving. Or maybe it was the offspring of a jockey's whip and a witch's wand. At that moment, I had no clue what it was and could never in my wildest imagination fathom what it was to be used for. The doctor clued me in.

"Okay," he said amiably, "Roll over and lie on your back for me. What I am going to do now is to insert this up your urethra." In other words, up my penis. "It has a light at the end that will enable me to see what is going on up there."

So there I was staring at this implement, which was about eighteen inches long. The tip with the light was slender, but progressively enlarged towards the handle. This was what he was planning to insert into my penis. *This can't be possible!* went through my now weak and frightened mind. The muscles in my back and abdomen went into a kind of involuntary contraction, and contrived to lift me into a sitting position. At that awkward moment, the doctor flashed a wry smile and said, "You should see the one I use for the guys I don't like!"

No doubt he intended this as a little side humor, maybe thinking I would smile or laugh and feel better by that "comforting" statement. At the time, it sounded like a purely sadistic remark. To my mind, here was a guy doing a drive-by on poor me, who had nowhere to run or to take cover. Putting one of his commanding hands on my shoulder, he encouraged me with some kind of hydraulic force to lie back again on the examining table while he prepped the instrument.

Gentlemen, guys, hombres, lend me your ears as I describe to you what happened next.

The doctor began to thread this "wand" up my penis, and immediately as it entered I felt a sharp pain. As it continued meandering its way up toward my bladder, a wicked, painful, and intensely uncomfortable sensation followed. I had never been tortured before, fortunately, and now I found it odd to consider that my first torturous experience in life was right here, right now, in a doctor's office in the name of good health.

There was one useful purpose to the penile examination: It totally obliterated all my memory of the previous examinations. No other thought or feeling could have penetrated what my mind was dealing with at that moment. In fact, if you had asked me my name right then I might not have been able to tell you. I was plunged into another world of discomfort, where all I could see were stars and blackness.

Fortunately, this did not last as long as the previous trials. Upon retrieving the instrument, the doctor announced that he had not seen anything wrong up in the area of my urethra and bladder, which of course was good news. I felt a tremendous urge to pee, which he knew would be the case and he instructed me to do so as soon as I got back into my clothes. As fast as I could move, which was extremely slow under the circumstances, I went to the bath- room and what came out was the frightening look of my urine mixed with blood. This was to be expected, he said.

Leaving that doctor's office, my torture chamber, I ambled away like a sad puppy, looking for someone to love and comfort me. When I reached my SUV, I had to climb gingerly into the driver's seat, instead of just jumping right in as I usually did. As I navigated the vehicle out of the parking lot and onto the main street on that cold morning, my Ford Explorer became to me more like an escape pod as I turned in the direction of home. I felt every bump in the road, but there was comfort in the fact that I was leaving behind the dreadful experience of these examinations of the most sensitive parts of my body.

When I reached home, getting out of my car was as difficult as getting in had been; the burning, painful, and unpleasant sensations announced themselves with new fury. I entered the house, labored up the stairs, and eased into bed. Without my intending it, my legs curled up right angled to my waist, and I felt more comfortable and safer in that fetal position.

The urologist was right when he told me that I would be seeing blood in my urine for a while, and that I should not be alarmed at seeing it in my semen, too. I followed his advice to refrain from having sex for about four weeks. When my wife and I did resume having sex, some remnants of blood passing from my penis made my semen look like cherry Jello. And that freaked me out for real. And why wouldn't it? Of course it would! Men are not designed to have blood leave them like that, but it was the only way to purge it from my prostate gland. My wife, a most special woman, understood.

With a course of pain killers and taking it easy, I was back to my normal self for the most part after those four weeks were up. The semen gradually reduced in bloodiness and returned to its normal color. This recovery was not without some untimely reminders of what I'd experienced, with discomforts that flared up after the pain killers lost their strength. But the pains gradually got duller and sank like a dying ember, scaling down until they finally were gone.

More Examinations...and Cancer News

So that is an accurate, blow-by-blow description of a prostate exam-ination and biopsy. Now multiply it by five, the number of times I had to undergo such testing. The mountain of pains were not the only things stacking up against me in the course of all these doctor's appointments and tests. I also had to deal with the psychological impact of this uncertainty about my health, fears of where all this was leading me, thoughts of my own mortality.

But from that psychological black hole, I reached out for answers in an ever increasing effort to put the whole business at rest once and for all. I was quickly converted into something like a junkie for information. On this road for answers, I traveled through three specialists to get their opinions. My personal physician was quick to give me all the referrals needed, and I became proactive in checking out those specialists as to their expertise, knowledge, and references from other people they had treated.

I returned to the initial urologist for a recommended follow-up round of testing, which you might find hard to believe after the descriptions of my time in his torture chamber. But I had no reason to question his capabilities as a diagnostician. This time he charged me one hundred dollars, paid for out of my own pocket, for Novocaine, which he used to dull the pains from the staple bites. The biopsy results, as with the first round, were negative for cancer, and I became very encouraged and thought that this cancer scare was definitely a false alarm and I could go back to my life. After finding nothing obviously wrong, the doctor ruled that I was suffering from an inflamed prostate and prescribed medications to deal with that.

But, to my chagrin, the symptoms I described earlier persisted. Blood tests showed that the PSA level continued to be elevated, and so we decided to get a second opinion. The second opinion, from a new urologist, concurred with the first. More medications prescribed for inflammation and so on, and those prescriptions I left unfilled. I had, at this point, little faith in those findings and the recommended treatment.

So I continued my search for answers. I didn't have any choice, I assumed, and if it took twenty biopsies to get the answers and to clear my head, that is what I would do. My next examination was when, you might say, the fish started to bite.

In my neighborhood was a nice looking building with a urologist's sign outside, and I decided to check this out on my own accord, no recommendations from anybody. I called the doctor's office, made an appointment, and asked my personal physician to send over the necessary referrals. Another biopsy: I'd become accustomed to the routine, but in no way used to it, as the pain, the discomforts, the bloody urine and semen were the same. Try as I might, I could never adapt to those.

This time—my fourth biopsy, performed by the third physician I had consulted—a-typical cells for cancer were found. An immediate follow-up was recommended, and I underwent a fifth biopsy.

The fish was on the hook.

It was a Friday afternoon, a sunny and bright day, when my cell phone rang and I was summoned to the doctor's office. "We had some cancellations," said the nice lady over the phone, "and wondered if you could come in today, even though your scheduled appointment is next week."

I told her yes, I could be there in half an hour. "That would be good," she said, "see you when you get here."

The first thing I noticed entering the doctor's office was that the place was, in fact, filled with patients waiting to be seen. That was odd, I thought, since there supposedly had been a lot of cancellations. But I didn't give it any further thought, and with the bait and hook in my gullet, I made my way to the sign-in window, and was called almost at once to go in to see the doctor. Later, it occurred to me that the business about cancellations had been kind of a ruse.

The doctor didn't want to delay for a week in giving me the news.

The news: The last biopsy indicated malignant tissue.

So it required five biopsies and prostate examinations to determine that I did, in fact, have prostate cancer. I had the answer I had been seeking for so long, though it obviously wasn't the one I wanted to hear.

Following his announcement, the doctor went over the options I had to address my disease. He strongly recommended a procedure called a radical prostatectomy, major surgery that removes the prostate gland and some of the tissue around it. I should go home and think about what I wanted to do, he suggested. I replied that I did want to think about it all, and that I would have to discuss the situation with my wife. "Absolutely," was his response. So I was brought back out to the nice lady who had called me in, and she was now even nicer and most empathetic as she went over some paperwork with me and recommended a particular book I could read to learn more about my situation.

By that time I was in pretty much of a daze, but managed to stand like a palm tree in a storm. Walking out of that office on that sunny Friday afternoon, however, I was trapped in powerful emotions of fear and uncertainty. I felt like a new bird, kicked from its mother's nest and unable to fly. Fortunately, it was just a five minute drive to reach home, and before I got out of the car I called my wife at work.

"Hi babe," I said.

"Hi babe," she replied. "What's wrong?"

Why she asked that question so suddenly I cannot say for sure. Maybe my "hi babe" contained some encoded message of worry and sadness that she could read. There was no getting around it: "The results from the last biopsy are in, and they say I have prostate cancer," I told my wife.

She was silent for a moment. Then, "I am coming home."

Sitting in our living room, waiting for my wife's return, I felt as if I was in the midnight of my life. The news of prostate cancer sent me reeling. The house was so deathly quiet that I could hear my own breathing. This was indeed a hell of a knock-out punch. *Mr. George Foreman, now I know how you felt when Muhammad Ali knocked you out in Zaire!* The "Ali bomaye" people were chanting was synonymous with the heartbeat I was aware of, pounding some kind of insistent rhythm in my chest.

The picture of my wife and my two boys, only ages five and one, filled my mind as I contemplated the worst. I knew only too well how very difficult it is for one parent to raise children, difficult for the parent and difficult for the children. My first-hand experience came by way of the separation of my parents when I was a five-year-old child myself. I knew first hand about the sorrow, the pain, and the disadvantages of having no father around. Though my father was alive, in many ways I was a fatherless boy. He wasn't nearby throughout the developing stages of my manhood, and I suffered by not having him to hold my hand and guide me through the fogs of youth, help me climb the hill of confusion and uncertainties that are part of growing up.

My children were so young. My wife was also young. The news of a possible terminal ailment was more than a blow to my head; it triggered off a gut-wrenching despair that I had not previously experienced. It was like a long night had descended, and tomorrow wouldn't come. Tomorrow was an elusive figment of the imagination. The gloom at that moment was as thick as mud and as stifling as soot. If there was ever a time I needed a silver lining in my cloud, it was now, and fast.

I suddenly jumped up, startled. Lost in my deep thoughts, I must have momentarily dozed off. But now I was literally on my feet and simultaneously filled with the profound realization that I must take action. Yes! This was no dream, but a stark reality that the man in me must deal with. I had to push back somehow, and fast.

My wife is leaving work immediately and coming home.

I have two boys to be a daddy to, and I must continue to be all that I have been and want to be for my dear wife.

So, up with this head of yours out of the damn sand! You are not some cursed ostrich!

I gave myself a fierce talking-to.

The doctor had said there were two other tests to do, I remembered. These were to determine if the cancer was localized, and if it was, the chances of nipping this thing in the bud were good. Anyway, didn't the nice lady at the doctor's say everything was going to be fine? These were glimmers of hope, and by golly, I would take them! I pitched out the "why me?" thoughts that were uninvitingly lodging themselves in my subconscious.

Spread your wings, little bird, you who have been kicked from the security of your mother's nest, or else you'll explode on the rocks below.

Spread your wings and fly.

Yes, you can still own a piece of the sky, if you just spread your wings and fly.

Sometime between my hearing the news of prostate cancer from the doctor that morning, and my wife opening the door and walking into our home, I arrived at a new sense of determination. There was, in fact, some wind under my wings now. I felt I could fly over this new obstacle in my life.

Chapter Three

Exploring Options: The Next Stage of the Journey

That is not to say that everything from that moment on was smooth sailing. And in fact, I went through a period of pussyfooting around before making the surgery decision. It took a while to get to that point.

For example, I briefly toyed with the idea that since prostate cancer tends to be slow growing, maybe I could just watch it for a while. At the same time, I knew that things had gotten a little different with me. In particular, I would say the peeing experience had taken on a new look and feel.

I invariably had to rush to the bathroom, and it was often very uncertain that I would arrive at the urinal in time. Let me put it this way: you have to start unzipping and reaching for the hose as soon as you hit the entrance to the men's room, and move faster than Quick Draw McGraw so as not to hose down your own garden. Compare that scenario to the guy who comes in after you, pees like a hydrant in one even flow, shakes, arches his back, closes the trapper, and washes his hands—and you are still there attempting to empty your bladder.
Now that is a stinker!

I will be eternally grateful to my personal physician, who stood strong in rejecting my pleas for Flomax. This is the medication that is intended to improve urination in men with enlarged prostates. In an attempt to take the reins from my doctor and see if I could drive this buggy myself, I had asked him to prescribe the stuff for me and let me try it. I had even brought up to him the advertisement's slogan, that my "going" problem was related to my "growing" problem. I had bought into that idea after being told that my prostate was "bigger than the average bear," but my good 'ole doc of Caribbean heritage said, "I am not giving you any such thing, man. Your PSA level is high and you are going to get that properly addressed."

For another thing, I just could not readily come to grips with one particular thought—the thought that surgery would leave me unable to service my wife. It was my responsibility and my obligation as her husband to pleasure and excite her, and frankly, I loved doing it.

Once, I explained such obligation to the nurse at my doctor's office, and she said, "You're right. Because if you don't, someone else will."

The wisdom of a woman!

I felt as frightened as a gazelle at a waterhole that had been pounced on by a lurking crocodile, As her words settled over me like an ominous cloud.

"Oh, but...," I wanted to say. "My wife is not like that. She's a cut above the rest, she is the pot of gold at the end of my rainbow."

I wanted to tell her that my wife reminds me of springtime when birds sing and flowers bloom, that she reminds me of summer nights and twinkling stars and the moon, and of the times I feel I can fly.

She reminds me of the peace that settles in my soul when her hands I can hold. That she reminds me of hope, the type of which I needed to cope.

Yes! She turns me into a poet, of sorts!

This wife of mine was a woman who cut through a thicket of opposition from friends and family to be with me. She had told her father to shoo off when he tried to convince her not to see me. She told him that her happiness, and not his wishes, came first, and that I was the man who made her happy.

A childhood friend of hers actually flew in from out of town with a particular crowbar of her own. The party this friend inveigled her to go to and the promise of the interesting men she would meet did not budge her. My wife stuck to me like a gecko on a roof.

This is the woman I had enclosed in the depths of my heart, after she had pieced it back together.

Yes, Miss Nurse, you can bet your bottom dollar, I am going to see to my obligation. All this I wanted to tell her, but instead I found myself saying in a calm and agreeable voice, "You are right."

The period of pussyfooting came to an end; the fight was on. It was now prostate cancer and me. I had also been given the good news that clinical tests indicated the disease had not permeated other parts of my body. Because my mother had no stupid children, I realized that if this was an opening I should really take it, and now, before the horse left the gate and it would be too late.

I had decided to follow the doctor's recommendation of a radical prostatectomy. Other procedures, it was explained to me, might not completely remove the cancer, while removing the host, the gland itself, would ensure that I would never have prostate cancer again. Without a prostatectomy, there was a possibility that, because of my age, the disease would re-manifest itself, and then I would be an older guy with it. I was persuaded that this surgery gave me the best chance of a quality life.

My wife and I had a long talk with the urologist who would perform the operation. My wife was the one who had read the book of information recommended to me earlier, and she now had all the questions. This urologist/surgeon seemed like a good fellow, who had condescended to be a normal person and an emphatic doctor.

So here we were in his office, my intelligent wife, who speaks eloquently with a Trinidadian flair, firing away with questions, while I sat, almost like it was my first day at kindergarten.

He first mentioned to us that he would not attempt the operation without blood available for a possible transfusion, since in this surgery, with the many blood vessels near the prostate, there was a risk of serious bleeding during and after the procedure. This presented a major problem in my mind. I was not going to accept anybody's blood in my body when there were better and healthier alternatives. Among the alternatives, we knew, was the use of blood fractions, derived from the four main components of blood (red cells, white cells, platelets and plasma), instead of the actual blood. Then there was hemodilution and cell salvage as surgical procedures to optimize the use of your own blood. One could also build up the blood through the use of iron to avoid possible anemia. We also knew that patients who are not given transfusions have a speedier recovery with fewer complications. Our research revealed that many major operations had been carried out throughout the country without the use of blood transfusion.

So we changed doctors when we could not be given the assurance that the Urologist who discovered the cancer, could not do the operation without blood transfusion.

Further research brought us to this other Urologist who has a reputation for not using blood transfusion on his patients. This urologist made us very happy when he conceded that "no blood" surgery "was better medicine anyway," as he said. He would plan to perform a da Vinci Prostatectomy, a method that he was trained on from its inception in France. The surgeon makes several small incisions, or puncture holes, to reach the prostate, instead of one big, long butcher gash through your abdomen. This method involves very little blood loss, less pain, faster healing, and also minimizes the otherwise lengthy hospital stay.

I had earlier expressed to the urologist my great concerns about impotence, and now, upon meeting my wife, he said to me, "I understand why you would be concerned. It's not like you are a seventy-three-year-old man with a wife of seventy-two. And you know what?" he continued. "Those are the guys with plenty of worries. Your situation is different, and your concerns are entirely justified."

My wife is a tall girl of five feet ten in bare feet, and a good six feet in heels. I remembered when I first met her, and not sure where this relationship was going, I tried to get her into the modeling business. She had the vital statistics for the career of a supermodel, and she became a favorite immediately to the people interested in training her to become a model. She turned her back on that invitation how- ever, and always told me later that I tried to get rid of her by pushing her into modeling. She was not altogether incorrect, as I couldn't understand what a beautiful girl seventeen years my junior wanted with me.

So yes, my concerns were understandable.

Imagine my relief when the doctor stated, "I will do my best to save the nerves." These run along either side of the prostate and they are what control erections. Nerves, indeed, that are vital to my virility. Another good aspect of the da Vinci Prostatectomy method is that when performed by a skilled surgeon, it typically spares the nerves, leaving them intact.

Now I felt greatly reassured.

Here was a man who appreciated why and how come I was frightened and concerned. Hail to that man, I say! That man who was my doctor, the one scheduled to do my operation. He had clearly indicated to me that he could understand my indignity and sorrow if I ever became unable to "get up and stand up" as a man.

That man understood that a plumber is a plumber, laying the necessary pipe when required. That he enjoys being a plumber, and not a carpenter or a mail man. Therefore, he was going to do his best to keep me in the plumbing business.

My wife was now happy and hopeful, and so was I. The only bad news, the doctor then informed us, was that I would be unable to father children after this surgery. "A two for one deal," he told us, "regrettably. A prostatectomy is always accompanied by a vasectomy." So he was probably surprised by my wife's response, as she announced chirpily, "Oh, I can stop wearing my birth control patch!" He was now looking at her rather quizzically, and I thought I could read his mind—he was probably thinking, here was a young woman who might be desirous of a child in the future.

What this nice guy of a doctor did not know was this:

About two years earlier, my wife had become prophetic, or maybe just responded to a dose of feminine intuition, and realized that it was now or never to get another child out of me. Immediately prior to that time, we had weathered the storm of a miscarriage, and I found myself thinking that this disappointment was perhaps for a good cause. Most men my age, I reasoned, have grown children. It didn't even seem selfish not to want another one, because I would save this new child some embarrassment from having to explain to his friends at school that the grandpa guy who picked him up and dropped him off every day was actually his daddy.

So for all intents and purposes, I was not going to go there. I remember trying to bat without scoring, but as my wife sank into melancholy and I realized what she was going through, I couldn't say 'no'. I did not say 'yes' either, but that wife of mine would get her man to a state where his actions clearly meant "Yes baby! Yes baby!
Yes!"

She then engineered a trip to Napa Valley, the renowned wine country in California. There I was wined. Then I was dined. Then I was wined some more with some of Napa's excellent red stuff, which I liked and enjoyed immensely, and before long all my no's and reservations melted away like butter in the sun and gave way to the "Yes baby!" mentioned above.

Nine months later our second son was born. He has brought us untold joy since then.

I couldn't let the good doctor continue to be puzzled, and I nodded to my wife to take him out of wonderland. "We do not want any more children," she said with a smile. And the doctor breathed a sigh of relief.

Chapter Four

Preparing for the Big Moment

When the time arrived, my physician promptly cleared me for surgery. Right then, I remember, he had a most sober and, I would say, "doctorial" look as he told me, "You're going to be all right, man."

On the day the operation was scheduled, I had to be on the way to the hospital by 5 a.m. I hardly slept a wink that long night. My cousin, who lived across from me, had come by in the evening to cheer me up and wish me all the best. I had even considered myself cheered up, and told him that if he saw my house rocking, he shouldn't come knocking, because that would be me taking a last stand, like Custer, with my wife. Yes sir, my last hurrah before they put me down.

This bit of bluster and bravado didn't last long. Who was I kidding? Absolutely no one but myself, as sex was the farthest thing from my mind that night.

In the morning, I felt a little hungry, understandably, since I had been instructed not to eat after a certain time the day before. My diet was to be only light liquid, and an enema had washed out anything else that was inside of me.

So there I was in the hospital, waiting to be led away. I watched the orderly prepare the stretcher, in the same meticulous way a good waiter prepares a table for an important guest at a top notch restaurant, and park the thing at the entrance to my room. At that moment, my unsteady mind took me to a scene on the African savannah, where a vulture perched on a tree limb was waiting for a wounded animal to die.

The orderly came over and said, "Your Cadillac is ready." I then hugged the three people of my support team—my dear wife, my mother, and a good friend, and told them I would see them later. This was the point of no return.

A week before that moment, I had been in the Bahamas.

Let me explain, again, how difficult it can be to put troubling thoughts out of your mind, even after all the questions have been asked and answered, after the right decisions have been made, after the appropriate steps have been arranged.

This was to be a soothing vacation—turquoise water, snorkeling, conch salads and soups, pristine sands, speed boats and island hopping. Top that off with some Bahama mamas and a beachfront view hotel room, and you can see what I'm talking about. Of course, the real icing on the cake would be my wife, who stood out like the most beautiful spring flower indeed.

Sadly to say, however, all of that felt like a last meal to me.

The trip had been designed and engineered by my wife, to lift my spirits, give me a break from the relentless cancer talk, and prepare me for the upcoming event of my surgery. But instead of the desired effect, I felt like a corralled bull. or maybe like a bird with its wings clipped, no longer all set to fly.

One concern continuing to occupy my thoughts—despite the surgeon's reassurances—had been that fear of impotence, the inability to get an erection, not being able to penetrate my wife, and her possible frustrations. That, and being laid up against my will, all felt like barbed wire around my soul. The idea of having to rely on Viagra or other stimulants, having regressed from a virile man to someone I could not imagine, was pulverizing me from the inside out. So at that beautiful location, I simply couldn't pretend that I was enjoying the vacation; the dark thoughts festering inside took control.

I found myself snapping at my wife for no apparent reason, and as smart as she is, she couldn't pick up just what my problem was. Again and again, she tried to pull me up from my descent, but each time I just retreated deeper into the hole, like a cornered beast. Finally, she burst into tears, described to me how she had carefully planned and paid for this trip. And this was how I thanked her.

Oh, how I love that woman! She clearly believed that if you're going to slaughter a sheep, you shouldn't let him see the knife. That's why we were in the Bahamas. Her sheep (me) was about to go through an unprecedented time in his life. This was her loving way of pre- paring me, giving me a respite, taking my mind off the upcoming surgery—shielding me from my fate, you could say.

I realized I should not and could not continue being in my black mood, and I started to explain to her my fears and concerns. My wife...my wife...put her arms around me as we sat on the bed in that hotel room, and she assured me that everything would be all right. "Everything is going to be fine", I remember her saying softly in my ear, and that I should not worry. The tough, hard core man I thought I was, he was nowhere to be found at that moment, as my emotions welled up and tears ran down my cheeks.

My wife explained that she could appreciate the fact that the surgery I was scheduled to go through was a mind-altering experience. I would lose an important part of my male anatomy, one that I imagined would leave me like a castrated ram. As I was staring down this dark barrel of fear and insignificance, she said softly, "I did not marry you for sex." And, "I will be there by your side. I will never leave you. Do not ever doubt my love for you."

She was a beacon light in my dark world at that moment, and the warmth I felt from her was greater than the warmth of the Bahamian sun. My resolve returned. I will do this thing. Like a good seafaring captain, I realized I had to move the ship from this dry harbor and put out to sea.

In the Belly of the Beast: Under the Knife

The orderly got me up onto my "Cadillac," and I was stretchered into another room after traversing a maze of halls, passageways, and elevators. There was even an elevator director. When we reached his elevator and various documents had to be looked over and signed, I thought to myself:

Damn, this is serious business.

Such a level of accountability!

Who do they think I am? The president or somebody?

Then his elevator, with him directing—i.e., punching in the floors—went down and down. This guy was in fact a bubbly character. I thought they had chosen the right person for the job, as he helped to relieve a desperate sense of finality. There was talk about sports, to which I joined in, and that helped me to feel that I wasn't being buried alive. We finally came to a stop and my orderly said to the elevator man, "See you later." It had been such a pleasant ride down that my farewell to the elevator guy was also a cheery one: "See you later, bro." He then wished me all the best. I said, "Thank you." Orderly and I wheeled off.

Through another passageway, and we came to an entrance with big double doors. My orderly hit a latch and they swung open. For one of the vultures on a tree limb, as I was thinking of things then, he was pretty nice too, and as he passed me off to the receiving person he patted me on the shoulder and wished me all the best.

The entrance doors had closed behind us with a unique sound, and I saw that my orderly had not gone back through them but went another way. So that door only opened one way, I realized. It reminded me of the preventive valve. I lay there taking in the scene and thinking that this was the belly of the beast, all right. A little

comedic voice inside said:

Boy, they got you!

Even if you wanted to make a break for it, you know you couldn't now.

Complete strangers were around me. I had expected to see some-body from my doctor's office or even the doctor himself, but this was not to be so. Instead, I was surrounded by unfamiliar faces. Now I know why a child so often cries on his first day at school. What a welcoming and cordial atmosphere it seems to be! But these are not your friends. What a professional and clearly proficient and efficient staff! But do you really want to be here? And those unfamiliar sounds and smells, they are not those of, say, your mother or your wife preparing a curry pot of goat!

No way, man, you are in the belly of the beast, and when he is done and excretes you, you will come out with one less piece of yourself.

Other people on stretchers were in front of me, waiting to be deployed like airplanes on a take-off runway, and I could recognize some who had entered the hospital with me. From the intake room to this station, it had dawned on me that I was the only one with no visible sign of illness, and also that I was the youngest. My mind wanted to

31

ask what I was really doing there, but, of course, I knew. I knew, even if none of the other patients knew, just as I didn't know what those folks were in for. I had taken the poison pill. I was there ready to have my prostate cut out.

Really, all I wanted to do was go to sleep, but thoughts like those kept my mind alert. What was taking them so much time?

Give me the smelling stuff.
Don't you want to see what I look like on the inside?

Let's get this show on the road.

Ever since arriving at the hospital that morning, I had been asked a lot of questions as the preparations got underway. Indeed, I was asked the same questions more than once by various people wearing an assortment of green and blue uniforms. They all seemed to be interested in my name, social security number, and date of birth, for the most part, and this struck me as extremely redundant, as all that information had early on been dog-tagged to my wrist. There could be no mistaking who this patient was.

Now, after I had been fussed over some more, a particular lady who had seemed suspiciously aloof came over and said, "Here is a mask with some oxygen, take some deep breaths of this for me."

So there I was. The moment of all moments, lying on a stretcher sniffing "oxygen." With not one familiar face to be seen, I felt like an abandoned child rescued by strangers. I wondered again what they were waiting for.

After the Operation: Coming To

"Wake up! Wake up! You've just had surgery."

Still a little dazed from that "oxygen" I had been given, I peered through the slits of my eyes in response to this voice and detected phantom-like figures bustling about. The sounds were different now than I remembered from before. I did have a desire to see who had just wakened me, but I couldn't really be bothered. It felt like too much trouble. But it was a man's voice, and the man said I had just had surgery. So there was the magic word. Surgery! And though I was still pretty groggy, it all came back to me like the emerging sun from behind the clouds.

As my mind cleared, I realized that the surgery was over. *Well, well. Wasn't I just sniffing that oxygen stuff a minute ago?*

You mean I have been through all that cutting and stitching, and my prostate is gone?

Now I knew how Lazarus must have felt when Jesus raised him from the dead. I was still a little groggy, but continued to be aware of activities around me, though I couldn't say for sure exactly what was going on. It was right about that time, and through my hazy vision, that I discerned the familiar face of my wife. I could sense that she was happy, and that was a great comfort. I felt her kiss, she said something very kind—I don't remember exactly what—and then she disappeared back into the shadows.

As I gradually became more alert, I mostly felt an enormous sense of relief that this was over. Maybe it wasn't so bad after all. It couldn't have been, as I had just had the best sleep of my life! As I lay there, I tried to remember the sequence of events, and the last thing I could recall was sniffing that oxygen. So that oxygen, it dawned on me, must have been the anesthesia. My roving mind rambled about here and there, and I thought how fortunate that I was not a virgin girl lying at the hands of some dishonorable fellow with that drug at his disposal. Strange thoughts.

Someone announced they were waiting for a room to be ready for me, and before long, I was on the way to the room where I'd spend the remainder of my hospital stay.

I was feeling just fine. My spirits were high as I thought of the new me. I had come through the fear of surgery and was now ready to fly off into a changed horizon unimpaired by prostate cancer. I had never been hospitalized before, but all the reports I had heard about the gloominess of a hospital stay and the unpalatable food didn't really matter. After all, the doctor had said I'd be in for only a couple of days. So I was, for all sensible reasons, chirpy and hopeful.

It was so good to see my wife and my mother. As I was wheeled to my room, we turned the bend off the elevator and there they were, along with the good friend who had made it his duty to be there when I came out of surgery. Their smiles and cheers lifted my spirits to yet another level. I felt the love and appreciation coating me like jam on bread, and boy, was I lapping it up. As my wife and mother poured it on, I winked to my friend and said, "You know, I intend to exploit this!" The chuckle that passed between us did indeed give me a new sense of hope and fondness for life.

Still sailing on this high note of jocularity, I observed that there was an extremely pretty nurse helping me get settled in my room. At that point, I found that all my normal reservations were unbuckled, no doubt due to the lingering effects of the anesthesia, coupled with my general euphoria over being done with the surgery at last. Obviously, I was under the influence of **something** when, in front of my wife, I started flirting with the very attractive nurse. I heard myself
saying, "I didn't know that nurses come so pretty and cute."

My wife, who was always in my club, immediately transformed her- self into the Head of the FOAFWPW (Feminist Organization Against Flirting With Pretty Women) when she turned to the nurse, pointed at me, and said as seriously as she could without laughing,

"Is he...flirting... with you?"

Then she turned to me with a look on her face that was half beautiful and half evil. The half evil proceeded to lodge a stare where my family jewels were kept. I have always had a theory that if a woman is really mad at you and wants to hurt, watch her eyes, and if they settle at the level of your most vulnerable area, get out of town!

I knew my wife had no intention of hurting me, so maybe she was just responding automatically to that feminine aggressive stance. However, if she had proceeded to squash the family jewels for this brazenness on my part, I couldn't blame her. I could blame the anesthesia. The nurse, who was not going to be deprived of this nice compliment from such a seemingly pleasant fellow, said without looking at my wife, *who was always in my club and who knows I was never a flirt,* "Wait until you see who comes later."

Later that night when the shifts changed, I realized what her warning meant; indeed, not all the nurses were pretty. It might be an excellent idea for hospitals to arrange for only pretty nurses to attend to prostate recovering patients, as this could be like putting flowers in an otherwise drab room.

The pretty nurse continued to make me comfortable in bed and proceeded to fix me up with the IV drip. This involves a needle inserted in a vein in your arm, which is connected by tubing to a bag of liquid that flows slowly into your body, providing hydration, antibiotics, pain killers, or whatever is needed during the postoperative period. The high that I was still riding led me to say, "I wonder how this juice would taste with a little rum added?" The nurse was fairly well tuned in to me by then, enjoying this chatty patient, I sup- pose, and like an old confederate she responded, "Probably not so good, you know. Plain water might be better with the rum, and this
is not plain water!"

My wife gave me an appreciative smile. "You're getting back to your old self, aren't you!" she said.

Yes indeed, things were looking up.

All this joie de vivre was not to last long, however.

Pain Management: Hard Lessons Learned

My jubilance was soon sucked out of me like water from the Sahara, and I started to experience a weird dullness. I felt like a Pepsi that has been left out overnight in an open cup, placid and minus all effervescence. I was scared. I was frightened. Something had eclipsed my happy mood. Something foreign. Something wicked.

And then another feeling took hold. My mother and my wife were the only ones left in the room with me, and the look on my face clearly had startled them. One asked me what was the matter, and I answered with one word: "Pain."

The pain grew rapidly, like an avalanche that starts from a little pebble and builds into a massive force of destruction, with me waiting in its path. As this wicked pain rolled in, I said to my wife in a pleading voice, "Call the nurse, please. I've got to get something for this pain."

She found and pushed some button and talked to someone. I think she began to panic a little too, as she started then quibbling about everything, the hospital, no one coming to help. She was worried and concerned that I might have to bear this on my own, but I replied, "This is a hospital. They have to give me something for the pain."

I said that partly to jolt her back to reality and partly for self assurance. One thing I knew for sure, or I thought I did in my misery, was that if they could not give me medication to stave off the pain, I was going to die. The feelings were completely beyond the scope of my imagination, and like nothing I had ever previously experienced. The closest description I can come to is that it felt as if someone had heated a piece of iron until it was red hot and then dropped it some- where in the vicinity of my bottom, my belly, and my back. Or in the middle of my soul.

During our earlier consultations, my doctor had told me I would experience post-surgical pains, and these would be managed by medications. So to someone who had never been in this situation, the words "pain" and "pain medication" were computed as referring to your average, everyday pain and Tylenol. Even if it was the pain of a toothache, which is no joke! I could deal with that.

I really was no stranger to pain. Once I chopped my foot with a machete and rode on rough terrain on my bicycle to the hospital to receive stitches. I sliced my thumb open on a tin can; stubbed my big toe without shoes on a rock, uprooting the rock in the process. I had cracked my skull running away from a pursuing cow. I have had dog bites, been stung by bees. The list could go on. After all that, I had in fact developed a high tolerance for pain.

So I was not worried about the pain after surgery that the doctor had talked about, mentioning it almost glibly. "No big deal," he seemed to convey, and I too, therefore, thought, "No big deal."

It didn't take long for the nurse to come, the same pretty nurse as before, though the approximately two minutes before she arrived seemed like an eternity. And boy, was I glad to see her. She wasn't the light and bubbly young woman anymore, however, the one who was enjoying my flirtatious attitude.

Now she looked as sober and dignified as a school marm. I guess you could say "a drastic situation calls for a serious nurse," or something like that. This time she did not even glance at me, and, ignoring my contorted face and my wails of discomfort, went right to work with morphine and Percocet. As she administered the medicine, my thoughts were:

This is a hospital!

They must have good pain killers here!

The morphine and Percocet did not work.

Somewhere deep inside of me I found the strength to dispatch my wife and mother for home. I had no wish to have them suffer from seeing me suffer. I had noticed, too, that my wife had lost her usual air of confidence, and it was now time for The Man (me) to do something about it. So I sent my two favorite girls packing. "Go on and get home before it is dark," I told them weakly.

That first night in the hospital was lonely and painful. After my repeated complaints, the medical staff made an adjustment to the medication that was supposed to help. All I know is that it worked for a short while and then the pains would return like a monster out of the dark. If I was asleep, they would pop my eyes open, flip me on the other side or jolt me into a halfway sitting position, in the process arching my back off the bed.

In the middle of the onslaught, I relied on whatever vestige of strength remained, or some presence of thought, to reach for the call button to the nurse's station, pleading, "Pain meds, please," into the intercom. The voice that left me was not me. No. Not the man that I knew, but the voice of a torn, emaciated victim of some war. The call, "Pain meds, please," could well have been, "Mercy, please!" Then I would slump back and pray that the nurse arrived before the pain reached its crescendo.

There were other discomforts.

I had been prescribed a diet of liquids to provide nourishment with- out any bowel interference. A tube—the catheter—ran from my bladder through the penis, to drain my urine. The end of the catheter emptied into a plastic bag—my pee bag—that was attached to my leg. When the bag was full, a nurse emptied it into the toilet for me. This contraption, though not as painful as The Pain, was most unnatural, uncomfortable, and as irritating as could be. My penis did not like it at all, and consequently shrunk so far up that I was ashamed to look down, much less have the nurses see me in that condition. Talk about a bash on the face of your manhood! I used to be "the man," or in the worst case, "a man" when just stepping out from the showers, but now I was not even like my baby boy's.

I had come to appreciate the fact that my urethral opening was fairly large, especially after the recent experiences with the doctor's penile examinations. But to have this tube that was bigger than any straw I knew anchored in my bladder, sucking out my urine, presented another facet of haunting and tormenting. In addition, blood oozed from one side of my penile opening—a natural reaction from small abrasions caused by my contracting muscles trying to push this thing out, as my doctor had explained on his visit.

Two and a half days came and went, and I was still in the hospital. This was not the deal. As I recalled, I should have been out in two days time, and I began to feel somewhat deflated and defeated. The pains continued their attack, and simply would not go away. If only they would ease up, I lamented, and I found myself wondering how long and how often I would have to dig deeper to deal with this as a tough guy.

As tough as I was, something tougher had gotten me. That something was The Pain and his sidekick The Catheter. The pain that made me weak. The pain that had me coiled up in bed and went straight to my head. More meds, more meds, I always asked for, but the pain still would not go away. And so I worked at keeping my mind focused on blissful things and happy times and my rambunctious and meddling boys at home.

Looking back now, I know that it was mainly the support of my wife that got me through. She would often call from work, asking, "How are you?" It was never really the question that was important, but the voice that was so caring that it caressed my soul. The love that she expressed in such soft tones was medicine in itself. She would visit me every day when she got off work, and lie down on the bed beside me. Before I made her go home—she always wanted to stay longer—she would tuck me in, reposition the television for me, kiss me softly, and say, "Bye. See you tomorrow."

She had become strong for me, I know. I would like to tell her that, if during those times she ever felt weak, that was me, borrowing from her strength.

Then one particular afternoon an angel walked into my hospital room. She looked like a nurse; she turned out to be my angel. She introduced herself, writing her name on the nurse's board, and in a voice filled with empathy and sympathy, asked me, "How are you doing?"

Normally, I have a tongue on me like Muhammad Ali in his heyday, but recently I hadn't been able to afford the use of many words in my speech. It had been reduced to a pitiful whimper of, "The pain." And that was my answer to her question now. This angel of a nurse, Mother Teresa maybe or Florence Nightingale, must have been apprised earlier of my plight, for now she said with some authority, "I am going to get you something else." There was a bright aura around her, and as she walked out of the room she left some of that radiance behind her in the form of hope.

That was the nurse who took my pains away. I learned later that she was a part of my pain management team and had seen to the change and administering of a different drug. Thereafter I often saw her making rounds about the floor; she would greet me and observe how much better I seemed to be. Whenever I thanked her, I was aware how inadequate those words were to express the profound gratitude I had for this comely phenomenon of a human being.

When she came back to my room on that afternoon, she introduced the new drug through the IV drip going into the vein in my hand. Immediately—yes, I said immediately!—a rush of warmth went to my head, and I could actually feel the stuff moving through my body. It was as if the thing was alive, launched through me on a mission to find and destroy the pain.

What manner of drug that was, though, I did not learn. One thing for sure: the hospital had it tied up and secured like my grand- mother's thread bag in her bosom. That drug had more controls on it than the space shuttle taking off, and clearly you had to pass through many checkpoints and final clearance before it was allowed to reach you.

Hop, skip, and take a jump, little David had defeated Goliath! I was finally pain free after days. Hope had returned like the arrival of springtime. Yes sir, I could see myself getting back to the party! If they ever get that drug on the market, I think the popular name for it should be "Little David."

We were now managing the pain. Another nurse explained to me that the way to handle the situation was not to wait until pain broke through the wall and then try to stop it, but to stop it before it broke through. That made a lot of sense to me. So because my mother did not have any stupid kids, as soon as "Little David" began to wear off, I would send my signal, and my own pain management skills became quite good. I did not wait for the medicine to completely leave my system, but timed it carefully. Just as that medication put one foot through the door on its way out, I would say, "Oh no, you don't!" and hit the button that summoned the nurse.

On the Road to Recovery

I continued to improve, moving forward like a baby on wobbly legs, shaky and unsteady at first, but marching on anyway. I had begun to sit up in bed, stand, and sit gingerly in a chair. Eventually, encouraged by the nurses, I began walking around the floor my hospital room was on. "If you want to go home," one of my favorite nurses, a woman of Russian descent, had said, "you have to try to walk and help your body get back on track."

I didn't want to let those nurses down, they who had cared for me so dearly, and most of all, I did not want to let myself down. At that stage of the game, I really did want to get out of there and go home.

On one such stroll, I hooked the urine receptacle, which of course had to accompany me at all times, on to the neck buttons of my gown to give myself more mobility. Otherwise, I'd have to carry it, and I wasn't too thrilled about holding my pee in my hand and walking about. The psychological advantage of being hands free of my urine was what I sought after, and now not aware that I had created some other bizarre spectacle. Also, though the pains were now manageable, there were still a lot of discomforts and I didn't want to add to them by carrying a load in my hand.

So there I was, ambling along slowly with cautious but determined steps, when I was pulled over by my Russian nurse. "Come here," she said, displaying a mischievous smile that I didn't quite understand. She proceeded to remove the pee receptacle from my neck and pinned it below my waist.

"So you didn't like my necklace, eh?" I quipped.

"No," she said with a chuckle, "but you know, it's easier to flow down than to go up, and we want it down anyway, not backing up into your bladder."

I imagined she would be telling her nurse friends how ridiculous I looked, strolling around the hospital with my yellow pee bag hanging from my neck, like I had paid for it at the jewelry store.

Those nurses were so nice to me. The Certified Nursing Assistants (CNAs) were no exception, and took equal share in my care and delight in my recovery. I do thank them all for the attention they administered with such affection. But nice as they all were, I wanted to go home, so bad. That desire had arrived like a Caribbean sun after a downpour, a downpour that put a damper on things both literally and figuratively. Just as so often the sun that had been shrouded by rain clouds pops open in all its brilliance, suddenly you realize that there are things to see, places to go, people to talk to, and the hustlings and bustlings of life continue.

And so I, suddenly, seemed to remember who I was, what I used to do, and that I had a family to take care of. A thought that kept kicking the back of my brains was saying, "You have no business here!" I asked myself, was it the kids I was missing? Was it the absence of all the people I was used to? Or was it this hospital room that caged me in?

As nice as everyone was to me, these feelings crept upon me so quickly they made me feel like a gypsy at a crossroads. It was not how, when, and why I got here; all I knew now was that I must move on. With this new fire in my soul, all attention was now geared to me getting out! Everyone, including the doctors, agreed that really, the best thing for me at that point was to go home. However, there were still some hurdles to overcome, and some had a psychological impact that only served to nail me down further.

It reminds me of how you catch a monkey in the forest. Get a gourd, tie a short string to it and put some goodies inside through a hole just big enough for the monkey's hand. Upon detecting the goodies, the monkey sticks his hand into the gourd and grabs the treats, rolling his fingers up into a fist that he then cannot pull out through the hole. Desire for the goodies is so strong that he fails to realize he is trapped, and that all he has to do to get away is to let go, open his fist, and retrieve his hand from inside the gourd.

So once again, my mother did not have any stupid children. I realized that what I needed to do now was let go of my constant obsession about getting home, and focus greater attention and effort on just what it was going to take to get me the heck out of there. In letting go of my "monkey trap," my walks around the floor became more frequent and deliberate, with a purpose.

There was another reason I wanted to be home, and it became more apparent to me on each walk. That concerned the sights and sounds of illness all around me in rooms on the floor. Having gone through my own experience, I could empathize with every moan and every groan I heard. I felt for those people. No one can fully understand your pain but you, but when someone has been through his own pain he can better understand. So when those people were moaning and groaning, screaming and hollering, they did not know it, but they had a friend in me.

However, I found that the environment of illness can have a negative impact on your soul. The doctors go home, the nurses go home, the janitors go home, everybody goes home! Except the sick. As the days stretched past the time when I was supposed to leave the hospital, I found that my aura was significantly changed from bright to dull, and there was a drain on my positive energy. This was another black hole pulling me in a direction I did not want to go.

I now became more determined than ever to get out of there before I did something even crazier than wearing my pee bag around my neck.

In my walks around the floor, I always passed by a huge bay window that looked over the I-95 highway. I would stop at the window and watch the cars and trucks go by, and that piece of asphalt looked as inviting as my wife on our wedding night.

Sleep came slowly now, as my mind became preoccupied with many things. There wasn't much to watch on television either, and often I would lie there just flicking through the channels. The bed had become increasingly uncomfortable too, suddenly as hard as if you were lying on rock, and all the adjustments that could be made to accommodate various sleeping positions did not help. Compounding that situation was the fact that both my sides had taped-up holes, and I was able to lie only on my back.

So I uncomfortably shut my eyes at night now. To get away from the torture I became the one to kick the rooster in his backside to start him crowing in the morning. What a night when you can't sleep and have to be up before the rooster!

One morning when I paused at my I-95 lookout, something about the lights from the vehicles and the street, the movements of the cars and trucks, some going south, some going north, gave the view a hypnotic appeal and its own aesthetic beauty.

That out there is the world of the living.

This in here is the world of the sick.

What I would give to be on that highway now, working my way north, towards my home.

A CNA broke my trance when she pulled up with a cart of gowns and linen, and we greeted each other. Making conversation, I found myself saying, "That is I-95 out there, right?"

"Yep," she said.

"Do you think they would catch me if I made a run for it?"

Both of us enjoyed the laugh that followed. My laugh was a little jerky, though, as the puncture holes in me wouldn't allow anything more robust. She, however, took a bellyful.

"Yes," she exclaimed between chuckles, "they certainly would." Turning to leave with her cart, she added, "That was a good one!"

I had to agree with her. Something like that could only happen in a cartoon—me gingerly sneaking out, clad only in my hospital gown, no drawers on, a tube hanging from my privates, and a pee bag strapped to my hip. Anyone who got in my way I could raise my pee bag and shout, "Back off!" like Yosemite Sam. Then the evening news would report: "Crazy man who had prostate surgery escapes hospital using his own acid pee as weapon." Of course, they would sizzle up the story by adding that "acid" to "pee."

As I stood there looking over I-95, those were my thoughts, and I blame them on a funny bone that I possess, which, if I'd been able to develop it, could have made me rich.

Physically, I was feeling much better by this time, and word had gotten around that I was walking about quite a bit. Earlier, the doctor had told me he was going to take me off the liquid diet and if I played a particular number—i.e., #2—they could see about me getting home. They had already pulled the bung from my side, a drain for overflowing liquid from my bladder area, and closed up that incision.

My mother came by to be with me that day, and the stories she told of the kids sent me into a state of frenzy, like a shark at a red meat buffet. The moans and groans of the sick, the hard bed, no sleep at night, no sunlight, no trees, no birds, no wind...and no children's laughter and noise. All this constituted the ingredients of a recipe for an emotional sour stew. Having eaten that sour stew for five days now, I was about to blow. There was a vice grip on my sanity.

"I'm getting out of here today," I told my mother in no uncertain terms. And by golly, I was determined I was not going to spend another night in there. The "ifs" and "maybes" that surrounded my discharge from the hospital on this, the other side of surgery, felt like no less than the trauma from an exit wound.

A Few More Obstacles to Overcome

After several days of only liquids, I looked forward to my first real hospital breakfast. I ordered scrambled eggs, pancakes, oatmeal, juice, and fruits. On its arrival, however, I realized that I didn't have much of an appetite, especially when I saw the pancakes. I am used to dainty looking pancakes, and these big boys—all three of them— looked like the kind you feed lumberjacks. Maybe there should be a law against giving such pancakes to a pained-up, weak, and recovering prostate patient. After some deliberation, I was able to force down the oatmeal, half of the scrambled eggs, an apple and juice.

A member of my discharge team appeared to see how I was doing, making it clear that he really hoped to kick me out of there, but first wanted to see me hold down a full meal. So the untouched pancakes immediately caught his eye, as if they were signaling, "Oh, look, he didn't eat us!" Like a little telltale. Some people would say like a snitch. I realized instantly that this wasn't good at all. Why I hadn't thrown the darn things in the trash, I don't know. "Uh-oh," he observed, "you didn't finish your breakfast." This remark was made in an accusatory tone.

Give me a break!

For crying out loud!

Don't tell me he's going to dock me for not eating those big, yellow, fat things!

I understood how strategic this fellow was to me getting out of there, and I knew I had to defend myself and fast. I had a stroke of genius. "Well," I found myself saying, "you didn't see that bowl of oatmeal that I put away."

I thought that gave me a leg up, but to consolidate my position I continued, "By the way, there is the bowl," pointing to the container sitting unobtrusively in the corner of the tray and of course obscured from view by the small mountain of pancakes.

I followed his eyes as he looked again at the breakfast tray. Then to complete the full maneuver, I added, "And also I had the apple. You know, the one that keeps the doctor away?" He was smiling now, and as I came out of the "swing move," I concluded, "With half of the eggs and all the juice."

As I rested my case, I looked straight at him with an impish smile. I believed I had him. I glanced over at my mother to see if I could spot the "well done" look on her face, and yes sir, the sign was there in a mother-to-son communique of half a smile.

"Okay, busta," my discharge team member said, "you have a bowel movement and you're outta here." Looking at my mother, I said, "I like this guy." He managed a smile, patted me on the shoulder, and walked out.

So two elements had to combine to get me home. Home sweet home, my own spot, trees, the neighbor's barking dog, ice cream truck bells, my rambunctious kids, and that mocking bird singing in the morning. At this time in my thoughts, I enjoyed a private and pleasant chuckle. The private and indeed pleasant chuckle was about that mocking bird. He had a special song that I had even tried to learn, a song that seemed to carry a message saying not to worry, a song that created such peace within. If that bird that announced the morning from the tree beside my window only knew how much he meant to me! If only I could talk to him now, I would tell him how much I missed him.

But about those elements that were going to get me out of the hospital:

The first element was me, myself, and I. I realized that I needed to tighten the reins of this horse and direct my body, specifically my bowels, to do what I wanted it to do. So the second element would be the functioning of my sphincter muscles, and I hoped they would not fail me for the pushing job ahead.

Earlier, I had been breaking some wind that I thought did not smell ordinary. Quite frankly, the odors were obnoxious. How my mother stayed in that small room with me without complaint, I honestly do not know. Once a gentleman told me that I was so ugly, only a mother could love me, and I guess her remaining by my side right then had something to do with that.

Anyway, I had business to take care of, and it occurred to me that I didn't have a lot of time available. Where was that oatmeal? Sure, I knew it was inside me, but when is it going to come out? I had chosen to eat the oatmeal that morning because of previous experiences in these matters; oatmeal had never let me down before. The apple should be excellent, too, especially since I had eaten the skin and seeds. Desperation was beginning to slip in here. Desperate times call for desperate measures.

Realizing that I had to take action, I called the nurse on duty and told him that I was bound up and I needed laxatives. He left to check on this request, and when he returned, told me that my doctor said no to the laxatives; no artificial inducing of a bowel movement was allowed because of all that had taken place in my innards.

I am not Superman. I had just undergone major surgery. I knew I could begin to heal quicker if I could be home. I have to admit that my determination was not fully charging at that point, and I lay back on the bed and closed my eyes in some despair at this new development. My mom put her reassuring hand on my forehead and in a mode of resignation, I started to think about getting some sleep.

Perhaps I fell asleep for a while. The next thing I knew was that I had an urge to get to the toilet. I should have been feeling good about that, I knew, and I probably was, but there was pain accompanying this urge. Weird pain. Anyway, I eased off the bed. I looked at my mother, and she said, "You want to go?" "Uh-huh," I replied.

My walk to the toilet was as brisk as I could make it, but I'm sure it had a striking resemblance to Fred Sanford particularly when he was having the Big One. I thought I had the Big One, too. Good grief! It had been five days, even though for four of those days I had consumed only liquids.

"This egg gotta be laid," I told myself as I slumped down on the toilet seat. Something popped out of me down below and I felt like a virgin chicken. It was painful. But I was happy! Now I could even cackle like a hen and tell them what I had just done. There was another thing—the smell. I swear that if there were city vultures, at least six would have been perched on the window ledge right then. That stuff was so stinky that not even I could stand it, and you know they say if you can't stand your own stuff, then it's really bad.

My next duty was to call the nurse and inform him of the recent development. My resolution had resurged like a crashing wave, the resolution to be discharged from the hospital. So come whatever or high water, I was going to be outta there like a Philly's home run.

When the nurse arrived, I told him my news. "What color was it?" he asked. I really did not know, probably being afraid to peer down into the bowl, but had I known they were interested in color, I would have found a way to determine that. I was tempted to point out that no one had told me they wanted color, but I knew that would probably come out sounding rather hostile. At that point, anything that seemed to be an obstacle I intended to jump on and obliterate, realizing that these guys held my fate in their hands and I shouldn't rock any boats. Hence my reply was nicely phrased: "I couldn't say for sure, but I can tell you the aroma could put a skunk out of business." Both of us had a chuckle at that. He then said he would see about getting me discharged, and off he went.

A few minutes passed and who walked in the door but my wife. This is a good evening I was thinking, as she did not yet know that I might be going home. As she proceeded to lie on the bed beside me, I laid it on her.

"Going home this evening!" The words came out with glee and full of childlike expectation.

"Okay," she said uncertainly, as if she didn't believe it.

"Yeah, for real!" I said.

She still looked doubtful, so I explained the whole deal, that I'd been told if I was able go to the toilet on my own, I could go home.

Right about then the discharging agent appeared, there to let me have the shinier part of his boot, and boy, was I glad to see him. "So, you had a bowel movement, ah!" he remarked, as if the matter was in doubt. I wanted to tell him that he should not scare me with that type of implied questioning, like some prosecuting attorney, but the chap was really all right.

"Oh yeah," I replied. "A big one!"

I was not about to leave anything up to interpretation, and at that point I was prepared to work this story like a twelve-year-old boy at a video game.

"Okay," he said with a smile, "you're going home."

Turning to my wife, I said, "You heard what the man said." Without replying, she immediately started gathering my things.

From gratitude and relief, I looked at that discharge agent and said, "Thank you." In one stroke, with the authority invested in him, he had taken care of all the "exit wound" injuries I had been suffering.

Chapter Five

Highway I-95...and Home

So here I was, finally on highway I-95, that road I'd been staring longingly at for the past few days.

After receiving some final instructions at the hospital and after a nurse affixed me with a leg catheter for the road, we had gotten out of there like a war pigeon taking flight. Heading north, my mother in the back seat, my wife at the wheel, me lying back in the front passenger seat like an urban gangster. The only reason for that position was because I couldn't sit up straight. Heading north, bobbing and weaving through the downtown Philly evening traffic, we had one common aim and one common destination. I was homeward bound. There should be a new song written, a new poem to capture the sentiments of that moment and myself.

This might have been the only time that I had not criticized my wife's driving. Usually, I was always telling her to keep her eyes on the road, slow down, hold the steering wheel this way as opposed to that way. Now, I was not in a mood to criticize. I was in a going home mood. So when she hit the first pothole and the jolt of pain registered in my head, I gently reminded her that I now have more holes in me than was biologically determined and felt like a punctured tire. Then I begged her in a baby's voice, "Please take it easy."

Noticing that she was coining a few words to respond, I headed her off at the pass by quickly blaming the city for not fixing the road with our taxpayer's money and the car for not being able to absorb the shocks better.

My weight was also crushing on my skeleton, and I wondered if my muscles had suffered some kind of atrophy. With taped-up holes in my sides and abdomen, for all practical purposes I looked like some specie reject from the spider family. The hose leading from what was left of my shrunken penis completed the bizarre picture I presented. But hey, I was heading home. Nothing else mattered. Even though the car continued to feel like a bucking horse and I had to grimace and groan from the stabs of pain, I knew that my wife was doing her best with what she had to work with. Negotiating the potholes and the lumps and bumps of the road was not easy, and she let out sounds of disgust when she knew she had inadvertently but unavoidably caused me pain.

I have been away from home before in my life, and for much longer spells, too. However, when I saw that house, the flowers and the trees that I planted and cared for, a feeling like that of a first passionate hug engulfed me. Now I could relate to people who had been kept away through no wish of their own. That was the big difference. It had not been my will or intention or plan to be away, and that is why, I concluded, the feeling of returning now was so overwhelming. That was why the sight of my house was so welcoming. I looked forward to snuggling up inside it like a kangaroo's joey in its mother's pouch.

So I was home and it felt good.

The last two days in the hospital had been torturous. The anticipation over getting out of there and the uncertainties surrounding the prospect had sandwiched me like an old car on a crushing platform.

I got up the stairs through much labor and discomfort. We were soon to realize that I couldn't get into my bed, however.

Getting into that bed had never been a problem before. Now, though, it presented quite a challenge. I thought that I probably looked like a cripple trying to get up on the back of a horse and not quite making it. All that didn't seriously matter to me. For all I cared, I could just lie on the floor, because I was home. It was my mother who then made the suggestion, to which we promptly agreed, that I should move into the guest room. In that room, the bed was much lower and I could get in and out much more easily.

My wife left to fill the prescriptions for me. She would also buy boxer shorts for me to wear, as nothing else was going to work with the hose and my privates. Boxers? I never wore them. Tried them once when I was a teenager, and they embarrassed me when in the presence of girls the apex of a tent would materialize in the area of my midsection.

Off she went to the pharmacy and the store. My mother began cooking, making some chicken soup for me, and the aroma started to climb the stairs and tantalize my nostrils. My oldest son came to lie by my side, while the younger one hung out at the foot of the bed with a toy truck that went, "vroom-vroom." Sunrays lit up the room through the glass French doors; my wife had pulled back the heavy drapes before she left. I was in bed, yes, and not the same me that had left it a few days before, but I was home, home sweet home, and felt so happy despite my limited condition and circumstances.

My house and cell phones rang often that evening as word got out that I had returned, but my wife, standing like a firewall, intercepted every one of those calls. Actually, I thought she was a little mean when she was shooing people off the phone, telling them that I was resting and could not talk now. But I knew she had put her right foot on the neck of this one and I wasn't going to argue, lest I incurred her wrath. And I knew for sure that she was only trying to protect me.

What a huge difference between my bed and the hospital bed! Cold ground was not my bed now and rock stone was not my pillow. And that joey kangaroo snuggled up in his mother's pouch, he had no-   thing on me. The icing on the cake was that I had two people caring for me out of natural affection. My mother's chicken soup was the best; in comparison, the dishwater they fed me at the hospital didn't even qualify as a distant cousin.

I had a relatively good sleep that first night home. My wife popped her eyes open from time to time to check on me, even though she is known to be a sound sleeper. Many times I had stolen her clothes off her and she wasn't even aware of it until it was too late.

The next morning on my road to recovery:

It was a summer day that I found to be so beautiful. At the same time, something was amiss. I felt rather cold and knew that I shouldn't be. Upon informing my wife, she put the back of her hand on my neck and announced, "You have a fever, I'm calling your doctor." What is she talking about, I wondered, never thinking I'd have to call a doctor about some lousy fever. Maybe she should go and see to breakfast instead. Breakfast! Doggone it! I did not really want anything to eat, realizing suddenly that I had no appetite whatsoever. My head sank back on the pillow.

"Okay dear," I said, "give him a call."

She had to leave a message with the doctor's answering service, and I was deeply impressed by how promptly his call back came. But in my cynical way I couldn't help thinking, damn, he must have thought I was dying or something.

A more sensible line of reasoning would have been that the doctor almost certainly had information I did not have, and it was appropriate for him to quickly check up on my status, and I should appreciate that. It definitely didn't dawn on me even at that stage how major my operation and the immediate aftermath had been.

In any case, his advice to my wife was to give me an over-the-counter fever reducer and to monitor its progress. The fever reducer worked, and I was able to eat a slow yet satisfying meal.

Well, what goes up must come down. That is certainly a true statement given the laws of physics. Similarly, what goes in should come out. Appropriately then, what you eat should come out, or at least the residue or refuse, according to the government of biological laws. So why was it that I could not poop! I was approaching the second evening at home, and I had not had a bowel movement since leaving the hospital. This was not a good sign. Little did I suspect that the euphoria I experienced at being in my own home once more would soon be dashed.

Let me now welcome you to the dawn of a certain era of my life that I hope I never have to repeat .

Goliath Returns, with a Vengeance

My fever had been coming and going, interspersed with sharp periodic pains of no mean order. Mildly put, they were vicious, and the pain medications the doctor prescribed were of no use in combating them. By then there were many concerns about my inability to defecate, even when I was using stool softeners.

The peeing part of all this was not a factor for now, like a nonstarter in a horse race. No! We do not have to worry about him! His trainer will deal with him later on. His not running was not going to affect the price of rice in China. Still hooked up to my catheter, the pee just flowed straight from my bladder into the holding receptacle. So not having to worry about the pee thing, the race to overcome the pain was on.

Around twilight time, I felt something like a desire to go to the toilet. But it was the return of the pain. I managed to reach the bathroom and my bottom crashed on the toilet seat. My behind muscles were as jelly and my weight was as dead heavy as igneous rocks, as a crescendo of pain hit me. When I first felt something of that magnitude I had been in the hospital and they had the stuff to deal with it. Now I was alone. Goliath had returned and there was no Little David.

At the hospital, I remembered telling a nurse that the pains were greater than childbirth pains.

She disdainfully replied, "How would *you* know that?" Which was a reasonable enough question, since I had not given birth. But I thought I knew what I was talking about because I was at the hospital with my wife when each of our sons was born, and my wife never hollered as I was then— though maybe it was just that she was less of a complainer than I was.

Now, my wife and mother appeared in the bathroom like genies out of a bottle. I grabbed onto my wife's lanky legs like I was expecting some special healing powers from them. The pains did not let me hold on. She tried to comfort me but couldn't, and then she disappeared. Later, I learned that she went to the basement to cry, as she couldn't stand to see me suffer like that. My mother, on the other hand, stayed with me for what felt like forever.

All this seemed so unfair. No one had told me that these pains would be so vicious. I also reasoned to myself that even the wicked person gets put out of his misery sometime. I knew I was not a wicked person, so why was I in this predicament? I felt like I had walked into an ambush with all retreat cut off. If I could summon up a tear, that was the point when I would cry.

To say it was a long night would be an understatement, because day-break seemed never to arrive. How I longed to hear my mockingbird. Maybe he'd be able to dull these pains with his song. I tried to concentrate on tomorrow, when I could get some advice from the doctor, but the pains ensured that such thoughts were elusive and gave no comfort.

I never had that bowel movement and only managed to pass gas instead, which is normally a relieving experience. The travesty of it all, however, was that I had to sound like I was being murdered from the onslaught of those out-of-the-world pains that accompanied the passing of gas.

Morning came finally in a fog of hope.

I hopped onto the deck through the French doors and a grey moon three quarters across the sky caught my eye, recalling the night when it ruled in splendor. Poetically, I wondered where was that silver moon last night to ease my plight. Why couldn't I, at those moments, have seen its light?

Adding to the night's excruciating experience was the fact that we would not be able to speak to the doctor before 9:30 a.m. If there was anytime I wanted to speak to a doctor, man, it was now. He *must* be able to recommend something to ease this pain. Adding insult to injury, we realized that today was Thursday, the day my doctor was in surgery, so he wouldn't be personally returning calls until later in the afternoon. Right then the pain just gained another ally to kick me where I sat. My wife, however, left a message with SOS pleas for some aid, assistance, or help for her husband, "who has just had surgery and is now having uncontrollable pains."

My doctor's partner called back as soon as he got the message. His call was reassuring, but not much help. Reassuring in the sense that we knew the office listened to messages, that they cared about their patients, and that they promptly returned calls. Not much help, because basically he had to wait for my doctor to leave surgery to give the go-ahead on any kind of treatment.

Fortunately for me, the bathroom urge had dissipated, but the stabs of pain deep inside my body continued to permeate my conscious- ness.

When I had first felt those pains in the hospital, one of the nurses had asked me to describe the intensity on a scale of 1 to 10. I had told her 20, and that was when I was under the care of morphine and Percocet. If she asked me now, I would have to say 50. And there I was lying on my back as the holes in my sides and abdomen were still fresh, making any other position impossible.

There I was with a monster devastating my soul and having nothing to leash it with, the prescribed pain killers and the stool softeners continuing to have no effect. I really needed a "bigger bag," as I was trying to catch Godzilla with a one pound bag.

And so a frantic search was launched to corral this Godzilla-like monster that was embedded deep in my personal universe and exuding its venom at will. The search took on a transatlantic/trans-continental nature, as advice from friends, families, and well- wishers poured in as to what to do and what to use to help have a bowel movement that would ease the pain. Warm prune juice, molasses with water, Castor oil, linseed oil, were among the recommendations. I availed myself of whatever I could get my hands on, but nothing worked.

Later in the afternoon my doctor called.

My wife apprised him of the situation and he informed us that the pain killers could be binding me up. He then recommended a laxative that was mild enough for my condition. We grabbed those quickly, my wife making another trip to the pharmacy, but again, nothing happened.

At this point I was not only desperate but mad. To disintegrate rocks, I observed, you need a stick of dynamite or a jackhammer, and I was almost ready to use those methods—except they would kill me. Finally, evening came and night fell.

There was something eerie and apprehensive about this night. I was home, yes. I was with people who cared for me and loved me, but this pappy was scared now. The premonition of a repeat of the night before was heavy indeed. I just knew that I couldn't go through another night like that one. Goliath was somewhere out there and he seemed to have partnered up with Godzilla, clashing their chains and stomping their feet. This was not going to be an ambush, but an all-out attack.

The warning was clear from the spasmodic pains that seared my inside. These were like the rain clouds of fear that grip the hapless souls of those living in a river's mouth, the thunder in the hills that makes them frightened. There is something dreadful about anticipating what is about to happen to you, especially if you know that what is about to happen is wicked and bad. And what makes it even worse is when you have no way of turning back the inevitable.

Given these circumstances and conditions, I was effectively skinned and tossed about like sheep without a shepherd. At this point—washed up like some flotsam on the seashore, like an abandoned babe in a basket—there was no David to slay this Goliath, not even Miriam to save this baby. I cringed at the thought of the looming night ahead.

The elder of my little sons came to kiss me goodnight, as he had been doing since I returned home. This evening, he lingered and wanted to lie on me. My wife had to nudge him away, telling him he'd see me in the morning, that I needed to rest and that I was not feeling well. I do not know what he understood about that. I do know that when my eyes met his eyes, I could see something similar to the look in my mother's eyes, something caring and sympathetic. As I watched his little legs walk away, amidst the spasm pains and the drumbeat of groans coming out of me, that special love engulfed me, the love that a father has for his boy.

The pains came that night. They came to take my life this time, it seemed. As the pain grabbed me with its tentacles, as it lassoed my feet with its cowboy rope, as it proceeded to hogtie me, I experienced an unparalleled feeling of helplessness and resignation. With it came a volcanic urge to go, and I managed to make it to the bath- room, doing what could be described now as a cross between Fred Sanford and a hop. Other aids along the way were the dresser, the wall, and the banister.

Everyone was asleep. A well deserved sleep, as they—my wife and mother—had fussed over me like worker bees all day long and into the night.

I felt a tremendous urge to bear down, along with dread at what I knew the pain had in store for me. At that point it seemed that all other senses were cut off. The pain then attacked in full force, and I couldn't stop the howling wolf sound that emanated from my soul.

I realized that I must pray to the Almighty Creator to take this cup from me. This was one torture stake that I couldn't carry anymore. I found myself asking God that if I had done one thing in my life that He approved of, and if He had a reward in store for me, could He pay me now by removing this pain? At that moment, I knew that I must breathe like a pregnant woman giving birth, and I continued to push down in spite of the wicked, awful, and relentless pain.

Something started to give. I felt movements, and then something like a cork flew out. The dam was broken! I continued to push for a good twenty minutes as stuff left me in squirts like a hose gun. With all my energies spent, I leaned back against the toilet tank for another ten minutes or so. Then I thanked Him for answering my prayer.

The worst was over. Thank God Almighty, free at last.

The most dreadful, painful, and frightening period of my life, as far as I could recall, had ended. And as I reflected, it was all caused from prostate cancer surgery. Of course, it could have been very much worse indeed, as if I had not had all those examinations and caught the cancer early, I might very well be on the road to dying. Now, however, I could continue to celebrate life.

I later learned that the pain was caused by air that was trapped inside me after the surgery. We are living in an atmosphere, I was told, not a vacuum, and so not all the air could be removed when I was stitched back up. That air had to find its way out! It worked its way through me towards the closest aperture, the anus.

Now, the anus area is where the prostate was removed. That area had raw nerves that were sensitive to every movement and every slightest jolt. Without effective pain killers, these factors had combined to form "the perfect pain."

A New Lease on Life

This morning after was antitypical to the usual "morning after" situation, which generally refers to the hangover feelings that follow a night of too much indulgence. This one was filled with joy and anticipation and hope, instead of fear, dread, and depression.

When I broke the news to my wife and mother, their bodies sagged as they breathed obvious sighs of relief. Even though the spasmodic pains continued, they were not nearly as severe as before. I was able to go to the toilet fairly normally. I chose my foods carefully, too, and ate as if I had had gastric bypass surgery, small amounts at a time. I couldn't afford the risk of being bound up and so I took all these careful steps.

A certain amount of discomfort from the incisions and from the catheter, still strapped to my leg, continued to hover like the dust from an implosion. This I could deal with, considering what I had just been through. So, feeling a great deal improved, I did what most normal husbands do, I started to irritate my wife. At least, that was what she said, and in fact, had remarked that afternoon, "You must really be feeling better!" when I told her to quit watching Judge Judy and go get my dinner.

This was the closest I had come to feeling my oats in a long time and the damn thing felt good. The little grin I flashed then earned me not only my dinner in a few minutes, but an appreciative smile from her, too. I didn't stop there. I continued jabbing away at her for a while, always holding the upper edge, until finally she said she was going to pull my "penile tube" that was strapped to my leg. Ouch! Now that was dirty and low! So like a pushed-aside puppy, with whatever tail I had remaining tucked between my legs, I left her alone.

This morning after the pain was also now the next morning on my road to recovery, and I began to think about the catheter—how they were going to get the thing out without causing pain. Right about then I was properly gun-shy of the slightest idea of pain. Pain exists to protect you, they say. At another time I might buy into that notion, but right then I did not even want to hear it.

In any case, the morning I was scheduled to have the catheter removed couldn't have come any sooner, as far as I was concerned. I had lived with that unnatural device long enough. With my wife at the wheel, we headed into Center City, me feeling a little apprehensive, but holding fairly good expectations, knowing that my member would soon be free from this harness. As my wife and I made our way towards the doctor's office, I almost felt like a kid being taken to the candy store.

In his office I was told to lie back on the examining table, and a very jovial nurse said she was going to pump water into me. "When I do that," she explained like a television chef, arranging her supplies on the table towards my left, "you're going to feel like you want to pee, and please let me know when you have that sensation." I said to myself, "Okay, Rachael Ray." (Rachael Ray is a vivacious TV chef.)

As she started to fill me up with water from the side aqueduct on the catheter, I immediately felt the urge to pee. "I feel the urge!" I almost shouted at her. It was a strong urge, but a strange one at the same time, considering the fact that it had been a while since I had experienced any urge at all, thanks to the catheter that was doing the

job for me. "All right now," she said, and whatever she did next caused the anchor to slip right out. Laughing, she said, "You have a baby!"
We all had a pleasant chuckle at her announcement. I should have asked what sex it was, but I didn't.

It *had* seemed like I was pregnant with the thing, of course, and only the nurse could have delivered it. And boy, was I glad it was out of me! My two-and-a-half week's "pregnancy" apparently had scared my member so much it had retreated into its chamber, like the head of a frightened tortoise. Frankly, I was embarrassed that this voluptuous lady had to be working with a couple inches at most of what used to be a full-fledged man.

My only consolation was that my wife was sitting next to the table. I reasoned to myself that she, the nurse, had to think that I was a normal guy, or this pretty young thing would not have put up with me.

The nurse continued about her business and presented me with what seemed to be absorption sheets. "Now you're going to have to wear these like diapers," she said, like a cartoon version of Little Red Riding Hood socking it to the Big Bad Wolf. I started to protest. I did not want to look like the old guy who seems to have poop in his pants because of those big diapers that he has to wear.

In the middle of my objection, she cut me off like a slamming guillotine: "Do you know we have to wear those for days every month?"

Not wanting to incur any more of her wrath, I said judiciously, "I feel you, sister," and with a note of finality, she replied, "Right!"

While all this was going on my wife was thrown back in her chair with a laugh that sounded like the cackling of a hen. After this, the doctor came to examine me and said I seemed to be healing properly. He then proceeded to discuss the ordering and use of a pump that was to give me an erection on a regular basis, for as he put it in these exact words, "If you do not use it, you'll lose it."

In order to flush out my system, I was encouraged to drink a lot of water. The only problem with that, as I soon discovered, was that I couldn't turn off the spigot when the fluid passed through me and was on its way out. This was especially the case when I was standing, as gravity then had its pulling-down effect. The water came out of me unsolicited. When people asked me how I was doing and I told them okay, if only they knew as I stood before them that I was peeing on myself like a ram goat! The nurse was right about my needing those pads. Weeks later I was still wearing them.

This condition, the doctor told me, would continue for a while, until I regained the use of my bladder muscles, and it was recommended that I practice Kegel exercises every day. These consist of contracting and relaxing the muscles that form part of the pelvis, and over time they help strengthen the weakened muscles that control peeing. I was also able to procure sexier guards with higher absorbency. How- ever, that did not stop the urine from soaking through and making me feel wet. This might not seem to be a very big deal, but I felt uncomfortable and unclean, and at times smelled like I was in some sad and uncared-for nursing home. I started disliking the whole business so much that I began to go through a box of fifty-two singles in a week .

Despite all this, however, I considered myself rolling through the valley like old man river, feeling very optimistic and positive, as I told myself the worst was over and behind me now. Those nightmarish pains had indeed gone, and with the removal of the catheter I could move about fairly without that stylish drag of my right leg. I consider that period as the watershed area of my experiences following prostate cancer surgery. Before, there were unabridged pains and discomforts. With the catheter gone, I could say I felt my wings growing back and I was edging my way again into the world of the living.

At times I felt impatient and wanted to do more, but my wife, especially, would remind me that the doctor had said I shouldn't be lifting more than ten pounds. She would pounce on me with the question, "Do you want to go back to the hospital?" Well, she wasn't going to be the one to take me there, she'd add. Now, whenever my wife gets serious with me over something and she has to verbalize it, it would normally be delivered in a thick Trinidadian accent. This time was no less so. And so I retreated into my corner like a corrected puppy, having gotten the message.

And then, some very important test results:

My next appointment at the doctor's was to learn the findings of the pathological tests, which would reveal if the cancer had escaped my prostate. I had effectively put this test and its results in the very back of my mind. Come to think of it, I hadn't much choice, as other things such as the pain and the discomforts of the catheter were readily available for me to deal with. Once again now, I was on the trail of concern. Notice I did not say a worry trail, as earlier clinical tests had indicated that the cancer had not spread. But this is prostate cancer and you cannot rest too comfortably too soon.

The visit was a good one, as the results proved negative. The cancer was contained. The doctor told me that if there was any news I wanted to hear, that was it.

Yes, the pathological test results were good. But other matters began to preoccupy my thoughts and had a powerful psychological impact. Specifically, what I had feared and what had scorched my vacation in the Bahamas became a reality. I was feeling better, the pains had gone, but something was changed. And this was as real and disturbing as it gets, when I realized I had no sexual desire.

The Next River to Cross

At that doctor's visit, and at this important juncture, with a clean bill of health as far as cancer was concerned, he returned to the talk about "losing it if not using it." I knew exactly what he meant about losing it. Before, I only had to look down. Now I had to look down and under, especially if my stomach was full, to see my "external organ." The good doctor mentioned that even though I did not have any desire for sex, I should use the prescribed pump to "wake up" my member from its sleep. He also pointed out that I could use it for sex, too. I guess in his profound wisdom he knew what my wife was going through or would be going through, and wanted to help me to help her. Let's face facts: she is young, and putting aside what she had said about never leaving me, as Spike Lee said in one of his earlier movies, "She gotta have it."

In my consultation with him I expressed these concerns, not so much for myself but for my wife, my dear wife. She and I strongly believe in not depriving each other of sexual pleasure, and that became a burden on my shoulders.

To such concerns, the good doctor replied, "You know, it is not only penal penetration that you can apply to satisfy your wife."

Having grown up in the backwoods of society, I looked at him questioningly.

He said with a wry smile, "Do you want me to draw you a picture with instructions?"

I smiled, and I knew he thought I got the idea. But poor me was actually so baffled. As far as I knew, there was only one way for a plane to get to its destination and that was by flying through the sky.

There were days when I felt down and depressed, and the sense of inadequacy would kill me. I usually love to watch my wife get dressed in the mornings for work. Often, I would pinch her on her naked butt and say with anticipation, "See ya later." She would reply with an impolite gyrate, and I'd feel a jolt down there, like a fish tugging at your line.

I could be Johnny on the spot, always. But now there was no answer from this sonar, not even a twitch, when I looked at her luscious body. Now I couldn't even say I was Johnny come lately. I recalled looking down one morning and saying to myself, "Darn it man, you are living with the dead."

My wife and I always had fun in our intimacy. We seemed to have an unspoken confederacy, strengthened by signals, innuendos, and looks that would build into the heights of intimacy. On one particular night she had sent one of those signals my way. Unbeknownst to her, I couldn't reply or respond. I felt crushed; like a jumbled wreck I lay beside her looking up to the ceiling. I could be appropriately described as a sick bird in a feeding tree. When I worked up the courage to tell her that I had no urge, she held my hand and a long silence followed.

There were not many choices at that juncture for me. The doctor had me taking Viagra, which had not helped. I was kind of happy when the erection aid I had ordered was delivered by UPS, happy as it might help me to soothe my wife, or so I thought. But mostly, I was sad, as I still was languishing away over the loss of my virility and for all intents and purposes, my manhood.

As I read the instructions and assembled the vacuum pump that was going to give me an erection, I realized and resigned myself to the fact that I was only doing it for my wife. Without that, I wouldn't give a cow's fart about anything. Mainly, all I wanted to know right then was that I had gotten rid of my life-threatening illness, and now that the pains were gone I could heal and go back to work.

The erection the pump produced was like putting a prosthetic leg in a shoe. The shoe looks like there is a foot inside, but there's no toe to wiggle. So the natural way for the shoe to bend and move is at best compromised!

I looked at my false erection and submitted that I had a ways to go. I wasn't done crossing this river yet.

Two and a half months after my surgery, I was doing well physically. Mentally, there was still that war going on, and I had to fight daily to stay positive. At my next appointment with the doctor, I was hoping to hear good news about the return of my virility. I really wanted something to stop the incontinence, too. That, with the erectile dysfunction, constituted an upper cut and a right. I was bobbing and weaving, even the rope-a-dope, but when it caught me in a corner, no bell seemed to sound.

A stick to cross the river would not help. I needed a bridge.

I wasn't going to get it right then.

At the doctor's office, as my wife and I kept my scheduled appointment and post-operative care visit, we learned that I was not among a certain ten percent of men—the ten percent who within a couple of months after surgery regain their potency and return to having sex properly and without any problem. It went further. I was not in that ten percent of men who did not have any problem with pee control.

The doctor expressed this news in a voice of controlled empathy and professionalism. But needless to say, my wife and I were not happy at all. We both felt a little like the bus had left us on the pavement, as the other passengers—that coveted ten percent—looked on.

The funny thing is that it was not as if we hadn't suspected this. We were only able to have intercourse with the aid of the pump, and there were so many problems with the incontinence. It seemed that what we were looking and hoping for was a crag of hope, the ledge where you put your foot for stability when climbing a slope. We wanted to be told that maybe in a month or so everything would return to normal.

But I, me, the Big Bad Wolf, whatever, was not in that ten percent!

The doctor, a nice fellow, apologized to me and mainly to my wife,

69

and she at once began to fire off some sharp questions, in a clearly disappointed tone. I was surprised when she candidly described to the doctor some "upstanding" aspects of my virility before the surgery and so, from her perspective and experience, she wanted to know: "How come he is not in that ten percent?" Before the doctor could answer, she had another question: "Did you save the nerves?"

This, of course, referred to the nerves that enable a man to have an erection, and which he had promised to do his best to preserve.

"I did save the nerves," he replied, "but they are damaged and have to heal in their own time." He almost surely had been down this road before, needing to tell a guy that he may have to wait out at least an eighteen-month window to regain his virility, and he added in

almost an undertone, "Every man reacts differently to the surgery."

None of this meant much to us now. Languishing in disappointment, we both realized and appreciated the fact that we had a long stretch on the road ahead, or on the road back, however you look at it.

My wife couldn't have been more disappointed than I was, or could she? It has long been debated as to who enjoys sex more, the man or the woman. I always maintained that it was the man, but looking at my wife's face that day, I saw an expression that was synonymous to the news of losing your mother. This was a serious personal loss for her, and I realized that I should never again hold to the view that men enjoy sex more.

There wasn't much else the doctor could do for me. It was now up to me and my body. He did, however, prescribe a medication to help with the incontinence and I guess, having observed my wife's facial expressions, from frowns to melancholy, he couldn't let me go with- out some stronger samples of Viagra. I really do appreciate that doctor. Apparently he dug deep into his bag to help me. If there was a spark of hope, we found it when he told us that one hour before intercourse was when I should take the 100g Viagra tablet, and then he added, "With stimulation"—turning to look at my wife—"you should be able to have an erection."

She was as unmoved as a rock and as stoic as a philosopher. It had been a long while since I had not been able to read her, and if I was reading her correctly right then she was thinking, "Yeah, right." And maybe she was thinking to herself that she couldn't believe her once virile man, who didn't even have to aim to fire, had come to this. Now he would have to clear holster, get ready, then aim, then fire?

It was no wonder that on the way home, we had only a terse and distant conversation.

It was going to take two united and understanding people who loved each other and who were patient to walk on and to complete the journey. Sometimes we might need a tow or to hitch a ride with whatever implement, tool, or stimulant we had, and yes, we would need prayer, too.

On the Road Again

We now came to the first time we tried intercourse without the aid of the pump but with the stronger Viagra, and this was in fact very encouraging. Another fundamental and encouraging fact was the results of my latest PSA test, which were good; the PSA measurement indicated no need for concern. The test reconfirmed that the cancer had been conquered.

I could feel the air coming back in me. I would rise out of the ashes yet and continue to be an indefatigable force. With a new fervor for life and a determination to win, I was on the road again, like Willie Nelson.

I continued with the Kegel exercises and could record a diminishing use of the absorbency pads. The sex further improved as anticipated, too, even though it wasn't that head-in-the-railings and wall-thumping type. And I attended a "Men Talk" session, a meeting that was organized by the American Cancer Society and that was greatly supported and encouraged by my doctor. The aim was to help men who were experiencing the kinds of problems I had. I was not disappointed. In this group, I found another bridge to the restoration of my mind and spirits.

I have never played professional sports, and so had not been in gatherings where men talk freely and openly with one another. What made this meeting unique was that we were talking also in the presence of our wives and other ladies who joined in to learn how to assist and be of help to their men.

One gentleman mentioned that he did not purchase that mechanical pump, because his wife was better than the pump. Another said he simply walks around with more money in his pocket these days, and that at sixty-five years of age, he's a happy man. When the time came for me to introduce myself, it went something like this:

"I don't know what I am doing here," I said. "I have no business here, I am not even fifty years old, but was diagnosed with prostate cancer."

My claim to this fame was seriously put down like a bullet to an old horse's head by the reply from one other fellow: "I am forty-one, and just had prostate cancer surgery." And his eyes welled up in tears as he began to tell us his story.

That first session I attended, which went overtime, was therapeutic indeed. I do not want to say it was warm and fuzzy in there. But it did cheer my heart when I saw that I was not alone. I saw men who went through what I had gone through. I saw men who had been afflicted by this stealth disease. I saw men who had fought back and who came together, not because they had to, but because they wanted to, in order to reach back and help another cross the bridge.

Chapter Six

The Second Stage: Incontinence

I was sitting down, but I had to stand up. I was lying down but I had to get up. Then I had to do the reverse of that again. That is sit back down, lie back down. This begins the story of my recovery from an after effect of Prostate Cancer, and the second stage of my journey.

It seems like I was playing the game of "Simon Says". You know, the lie down get up, sitting down standing up. But that was my experience as I coped with the second surgical procedure to become "normal again" and as I climbed out of the swampy morass of prostate cancer.

The first procedure, the Prostatectomy, the complete removal of my prostate gland along with some of my manhood and testosterone, was an ordeal from which I had adequately bounced back. However the marsupial agility of which I was accustomed to was severely lacking, and I could not accept that as normal.

In this case, to be normal again meant I had to hit all three bases. That's right! three bases were in this game that must be hit.! The first base and definitely the most important base is getting rid of the cancer. All subsequent tests and analysis had proved that we were successful in covering that base.

The second base which is highly esteemed in the world of men and of paramount importance to women is the ability to have an erection. That blessing was bestowed on me in fine manner. There were scary moments though, where I felt like something buried alive, from the lack of sensitivity in that department, when nothing worked.

The third base to be covered was that of incontinence, an inability to control the urine flow. That, for me, is where the second hill begins.

The urine flowed out of me like an overturned bucket.
Now this urine, mind you, was not that of a baby, but that of a grown man now fifty one years old. A fifty one year old man such as me may drink a beer, when thirsty, and because we are 70% water we are encouraged to drink as sufficiently to flush our system. A man of my age is allowed of course, to have that adult drink, drink coffee, tea sodas, juice as the case may be. When the biological process is complete and the liquid has to pass through you it can be putrid and smelly.

My urine was no less putrid and smelly.

After almost 18 months of this incontinence, and for all practical purposes peeing on myself, I came upon the realization that this was not stylish any more, than a sheep baying at the moon.

My two year old son was in a much better position than me. Here he was being trained to say when he wants to pee and allow us to put him on the training potty without him having to wet himself. His urine was also nice and fresh (as baby pee should). Little did my baby boy know that at this stage and under the circumstances his old man was jealous, and wished that his urine could be as fresh and nice as his.

At this point too, I remembered being told by my grandmother when I misbehaved as a boy, that I must be *smelling my pee.* As the time went by and as I entered the passage of manhood, she would have to use that term often, and embarrass me real good in the process.

Oh yes grandmother! I am *smelling my pee*! It took all but of fifty one years, but I am smelling my putrid and reeking pee!.

My passage to manhood however was without *smelling my pee*. I never even wet the bed like my sister, and never had to wash bed sheets as punishment as she had to. It took me 50+ years to smell my pee as a result of Prostate Cancer and as a result of the male pads that I had to wear due to incontinence!

So 18 months into this experience, enough was enough.
As loving and understanding as the lady who is my wife was, enough was enough for her too.
Whenever we lay down on clean sheets she had to wash them along with various towels, the next morning before going to work. As happy and joyful as we were that we had scored this second base of overcoming the impotence, the inconvenience of having a busted pipe with us in bed became too much.

Enough is enough!
My good doctor and Urologist had also agreed that "enough was enough" and something needed to be done about this. The Kegel exercises had not worked, the prescribed medications had not worked either.

As thorough as my doctor is he wanted *three out of three*. He was determined to find me a way to cover third base and to rid me of this Ram goat behavior, of peeing on myself.
With his determination and my willing attitude we embarked on a course to efface incontinence from the map of my life.

As he was winding up to make this pitch I blew a whistle like:
"Can we try some other medication?"
"No!" He said from the perch of his doctor's *high chair*
"We have tried enough meds and after 18 months if they have not worked, surgery is your other option", he concluded.

"Surgery again" I thought as the realization hit me.

To be cut again, to be wounded again, to be lamed up for another spell, were the other waves that bashed my mind.

I still thrive some, on the thought, that surgery should be my last resort. Also from some earlier stage of my life, the order of the day was that you do not take cut, but instead you give cut. So this cutting thing really do not sit well with me.

But this was my doctor, a man I came to call friend, and I guess from his crow's nest perspective there was no other rescue boat on my horizon.

My wife and I had now enjoyed ten years of marriage at this juncture of my life. One contributor to our success was selflessness. I realized at this point that even if I could turn up my nose and bear it she shouldn't be expected, to grin and bear it. Yes! Enough was enough!

If I hadn't known better I would think my doctor was a military commander. His young boyish look was no compliment to his demeanor when in military fashion he whisked me from hesitancy to decision and on my way to the appointment with my next knife.

I wasn't going to go so easily though and still lingered in the rear like a yellow–belly on the frontline. So, with my heels in the dirt while the taut rope of decisiveness was around my neck, I said to him,
"Hey doc?"
to which he answered, "Eh-hem"
"This is not going to affect my sex life?!" I kind of stated, kind of asked.
"NO!" he almost shouted. 'As a matter of fact it might make it better".

I could certainly breathe better after that answer. My wife and I had worked with special care and attention to get my feet back in the stirrups and we couldn't afford to be thrown by this mule of erectile dysfunction again.

My doctor then proceeded to describe the procedure and how it worked.

"We are going to put a *sling* inside the bladder area" he said.

He did not know it, but the good doctor lost me then. For some reason, sling and black men do not go well together. It has a connotation of a *strange tree bearing strange fruit.* The fact that my doctor is white certainly did not help my flashback to a particular era in black history. However, I know beyond the shadow of a doubt, that there is not one prejudice bone in his anatomy. To me this man was a friend, as I said before. But he studied medicine and I studied history and the historical side of things for some strange reason took root at that moment, albeit briefly.

I came out of this one through some port in my mind that takes me back to Jamaica where there is a motto that says "Out of Many One People". Yes, out of many races including whites everybody is one, and so there is *no problem mon.* As I came back into the picture I was appreciative of the fact that I was black, as the drainage of blood from my face would have been obvious, exposing my moment of fear.
I hate showing fear. It is a long known fact that fear magnetizes the worst to you. So as far as I am concerned the good doctor did not read my poker face and he was none the wiser.

Proceeding he said, "We are going to make the initial appointment for you now…with my partner".
It was then that I find myself saying "What?!".
I did not know of any partner. Probably what I meant to say is that I did not care about any partner.
This man, whatever he did, had made me trust him. In the surgery business it has been said that the assigned surgeon sometimes passes you onto his trainee doctor to practice on you. When you are under the drug that makes you almost dead, you cannot object to this student in a training exercise on you. What some people do is to have the

surgeon sign an affidavit agreeing and stating that he would be personally responsible for, and will be doing the surgery himself.

This indeed makes a lot of sense as certain delicate operations should only be done by the experts. Until the trainee has operated on a certain number of pigs (who have the closest anatomy to humans) and until he has operated on a particular threshold of humans he is not an expert. You might not be The President but you should insist that the knife should only be in the top guy's hand. That principle saved President Reagan when he was shot. Therefore this is a word to the wise.

As stated I trust my doctor and have a general belief in doctors as "aids", for want of a better term, to a healthy society. On a whole though, I do not trust them. That is why I have been going to my primary physician for over twenty years. And by golly! he is not the most personable fellow nor does always exercise good manners, but I have come to know and believe in him.

Suffice it to say then that this change of captains in the middle of this storm was not sitting well with me.

I needed to explain to my doctor that a storm has a front piece, the calmer eye, and an equally devastating piece at the back. If we had weathered the front piece which was the trauma of the prostatectomy, and now going through the relative calm of the eye, there was no way that I was going to let a doctor that I am not accustomed to, navigate this crucial and very important leg of this journey. Indeed, I want to weather the full force of this storm of my life, and not to be washed away by a surprising end-force wind.

I felt my doctor was burning the adoption papers and for a moment I returned to the world of my reeking self and thought that it was my private world of course, and maybe if I tried, I could live with this. I could feel the 'throw in the towel face' pasting itself on my features as I contemplated this.

Then, from the right corner of my consciousness looms the face of my wife. A thought then anchored in my belly that if there was one woman in the world who does not deserve a man who pees on himself and smells like a ram goat, it was she.

Resignedly I look up at the doctor. I knew there was no poker face this time and he had apparently read me like one of his x-rays.

My doctor then took time out to explain to me like a pupil at his feet why his partner was the best for the job. That he was good, and that he would take good care of me. And above all, that he was definitely the specialist in this area (*of slinging people up*). I was assured that he was the best in this neck of the woods that is Southeastern Pennsylvania.

So it came back to me; the recognition, the re-enlightenment, I felt different this time like some scummy dross was removed from me and the sun come shining through. I knew then that I must go the extra mile in my journey with prostate cancer, because…enough was enough.

The News And My Wife

When I walked out of the doctor's office that morning, as I continued my post prostatectomy journey, it was another important morning of my life.

There was something afoot here. I couldn't shrug the feeling. With my decision to go ahead with this, I was now experiencing the mixed sentiments of dread and gleeful anticipation. For sure, the dread of something going radically wrong, and the glee of getting back my life.

I had just signed up for another surgery, in less than 18 months. That meant another deathful or deathlike sleep brought on by general anesthesia, and the uncertainties associated with it.

The procedure was going to be simple the doctor said, and I will be in and out in a day. But then came the sinking thought in a most uninviting way like some obnoxious party crashers: *some people go in for simple procedures and do not come back out.*

Indeed this was my bear trap! I had stepped onto it and it goes "Clamp!" around my legs. The bear trap has associations with the cobra in my path! For crying out loud... I had stepped on him too and the venom from his bite has raced to my nervous system, and I felt trapped and paralyzed. There was no turning back now, that I was quite aware of. However, those were the fears that gripped me and held down my head in dread and doubt.

Till today no one knew this, but I thought that something dreadful was ominous. I had gotten through the first surgery without any problems as such. However, my gut feelings were that it may not be the same this second time around.

But what about my wife, the woman that I would do anything for? The woman who if she turns in her sleep wakes me? The woman who, when sad stops my sun from shining? You see, I could be normal again and when we lay down again we could have the warmth that we are accustomed to. When we lay down it could be like the warmth of a summer camp fire instead of the wetness of a leaking roof. This was the gleeful anticipation... and by golly! It tipped the scale in the right direction.

I was going to hold onto this positive feeling. Not only did it make me feel better, but deep down I knew I had made the right decision. I couldn't wait to discuss this with my wife. It also dawned on me that I had made the decision to go ahead with this without talking it over with her.

It did not even feel wrong as it probably should. Compare that to the times when I made decisions without consulting with her, and how bad I felt after. Especially when they did not turn out right. She had suffered silently enough. That, I knew. This, I confirmed to myself, was my decision to give her back the man she married. She deserved much more than to be living with a form of an eighty year old man at fifty something. Yes! I was not the coward of the county and as I began to feel my hands clasping on the controls of my life once again, I knew I must fight as a man. I reminded myself that I had two out of three. There was only this final wagon to be hitched up to my train, and I could resume my roll over the prairie, with my beautiful wife at my side. We could smell the roses once again and listen to the raindrops on the window pane.

That evening, when my wife came home from work, we sat in the love seat and I began speaking.

I reiterated what I was going through and my dissatisfaction with this way of life.

I also recalled to mind that my doctor had earlier told me that if the incontinence condition had not improved, he could have it stopped or improved surgically.

I told her then, what was my decision; to go ahead with the surgery and get it over with.

I also told her that I had an appointment with another doctor already that was a partner in the practice, that I was convinced he could take good care of me, and that everything should be okay.

My wife's eyes then lit up, her chest went up, while she simultaneously squeezed my hand,…then… her chest went down again.

This was the release from the bear trap…the antidote I needed for that snake poison of doubt, uncertainty and fear.

I was glad that I made the decision on my own so that I could present it as some kind of gift to her. I could sense her expectation and anticipation of relief. Yes! One day and soon, she will unwrap this package and will not want to return this gift. The gift of me to her, as she had known, and not some smelly incontinent man.

"I love you" She said.

I took her in my arms then and embraced her in a passionate hug.

Chapter Seven

The Beginning of the End

And just like that another period of my life had come into focus. Sometimes these periods can come down crashing with devastating force, fortunately for me that was not the case. The moment had come from sometime ago and somewhere earlier in this development, when I realized that nothing had worked to address the incontinence. That time was about half way through the 18 month period when I woke up every day looking for a change, but no change would come.

So I puffed up my chest like a cock pigeon and stepped out on the ledge. I was proud of myself too, that I had not skylarked around. And after overcoming those initial and peculiar feelings of the sling, and a strange doctor, I knew I had arrived at the beginning of the end.

This was the beginning of the end of a smelly, yucky, experience that had overshadowed every facet of my life. I had been effectively cocooned in that private world of stench and unpleasantness. I was never without the protective male pads. They were supported by lock straps in my jockey shorts or by themselves in a more tightly fitted brief. I was not even amused by the new side-elevation view that they gave me. This was even more pronounced when unable to change the pad for some reason or the other and it would fill up and expand. In fact it only reminded me of something like a false buttocks that some women who are trying to achieve a bigger derriere wear.

How could I live with this condition really? The putrid smell was so obvious to me even when there wasn't any. I feared something as natural as sneezing to clear my nostrils, as this would invariably release a squirt gun action in my pants. This could even result in certain embarrassment for me depending on the saturation level of the pad and the color of my slacks, where it could become obvious to every one that my crotch was wet.

On one such occasion, I was hanging out with a friend and his wife at their house. I was only about a mile from my house and didn't bother to take a spare pad. We were laughing and talking and I had enjoyed a cup of black coffee in the process. Now all of this could be construed to be normal activity for most people. For me though, this turned out to be my first taste of public embarrassment, seen to, by incontinence. That day I wet myself very badly. I was further flung into shame when I had to wear my friend's underwear, supported by one of his wife's sanitary napkin, back to my place.

Another occasion of a depressed and sad moment for me happened when my family was visiting with two other families.

Traditionally we had always done this, sharing or rotating venues and the association and socialization that we had was something we always looked forward to.

It was our time to make the trip.
I had a call from the host that the grape's cap was removed and that she was breathing expectantly. To translate he had opened the bottle of wine so that it would be well breathed by the time of my arrival. Now I like emptying a bottle you see, especially when the ambience is contributed to by great friends, good conversations and a good meal. From all perspective, this was going to be a great time. It would have been too if my private urinary incontinence world had not intruded. Every glass of wine, gully-washed through me like Hurricane Katrina was its mother. The absorbency of those pads could not save me, and

the overflows and runoffs exploded in my crotch like a mad river in spate.

I was soon to loose my social equilibrium and was lost to the warmth of the gathering. My friends would not have known this fact: that this was the first time I was with them but was not there.

Of course my wife noticed that something was wrong, and her search for answers with her eyes to my eyes, were confirmed by my message... a squeeze from me onto her hand. We knew we had to leave then, and under the cover of darkness where I could hide the shame of my wetness, I was able to save face as we slipped away, and drove home.

There was another occasion when I was accosted by this incontinent scenario. This was when I had to meet with my lawyer and a friend to discuss some business matters.

After we ground through the meatier matters on the agenda, we came up for air and the jokes began to be cracked. I remembered starting to laugh when the gush got me. Although I was wearing a pad, (of course I couldn't leave home without it) the realization was enough to put my lights out.

As my psyche left the scene, my friend asked if I was okay. Okay? How did he know I was not okay? was my immediate thought.
Now I knew I couldn't even hide behind the wall anymore! Every body and his mother have x-ray vision! Incontinence was messing with my existence! I realize I couldn't even look at the fellow but did shake my head affirming that I was okay, when I really wasn't.

The beginning of the end had long been forthcoming. I knew that I couldn't live like this any longer.
Any other thought or claim that I may have had, had no grounding or foundation, and yes, I may have thought I could live with this, but that

would only have been periodic, in moments of insanity, and fleeting at its best.

Such thoughts could have been more appropriately described as the strands of foolishness that were preventing me from the exuberance and the normalcy of life that I deserved.

I could see clearly now that this was not just a bug on my windshield, but a boulder in my way. This is a prisoner that I will not take. This condition of incontinence as a result of the prostatectomy, had to go.

Chapter Eight

Second Dance with Surgery

The time had now come for my consultation with my *sling specialist*. I cannot say that everything went smoothly. I had arrived for a 9:30 appointment, was on time, and was never seen until almost three hours later.

This did not help my idiosyncrasies about a new doctor. Here it was like you going in for that first kiss and the girl did not pucker up at all. Sitting down in that waiting room bothered me like a bugging fly. I wanted to leave really bad, or at least reschedule the appointment. My stomach reminded me that I had not even had a cup of anything and the mixture of madness and hunger had built up into a fine sour gut of emotions indeed.

As disgruntled as I was, I did not leave, but instead called, guess who, my wife. Now my baby got mad and was even madder than me. She started to tell me what I should do from what I shouldn't do, to get them to see me. She was so mad that I found myself calming her down. She knew I would clear a forest for her and I guess I should know she would burst through a wall for me too.

This was another of those occasions that I realized that my wife and I had really become one. She felt my frustration, or more appropriately sensed it and so the questions burst from her like laser light, poignant and feisty. Who do they think they are anyway? Do they know people have things to do? Have you talked to the office manager? I started to ooze my own ingredients into the mix by saying "And I haven't even eaten anything from this morning". Bolstered up by her I got on my feet and was approaching the manager's window to confront somebody, when my name was called from somewhere down the passage towards the intake rooms. Turning, I saw a nurse with a manila folder in her hand.

I informed my wife of this development who made another assertion of their unacceptable tardiness with the instruction that I should call her as soon as I was finished. I put the cell phone away and walked towards the nurse. I was kind of glad too that I had not thrown this switch into reverse, as I was about to.

Finally, in my second dance with prostate surgery, they seemed to have changed the tune from that scratchy introduction to a smoother waltz.

This was when I met the partner of my Urologist.

The dude was cool if not smooth. A couple minutes with him and I had totally forgotten the whole introduction. He jumped onto the stage with his suave self and presented a rainbow of doctor's manners, skills and empathy, that I find hard to believe he would have learned in schools. He was built like Lance Armstrong, debonair by character and had only the white coat to authenticate him as the doctor or a doctor. His commanding presence was always announced by the moaning of the tile underneath his heavy soled black shoes, as he lifts them up and puts them down like government boots, moving from room to room, and patient to patient.

I am certain that I was not the only one who was incensed by the long wait to be seen. As a matter of fact there were audible expressions of disgust in the waiting area from almost everyone. However, everyone was probably mesmerized or hypnotized by this doctor dude, that no one said anything or expressed anything to him, about the shoddy operation of herding everyone in here at the same time for the same appointment. This sharp fellow, this doctor dude, like a Gestapo with a smile has doused that for sure!

"Mr. Martin!?" he announced on entering the room I was waiting in.

"Hey doc" I said waiting for him to strike the next pose, and respectfully recoiled myself into a dignified ball in the patient's chair.

In my previous surgery, at this juncture I felt like a dropped off child on his first day of kindergarten. But now, it was more like college stuff. I was aware of the course I was taking and was ready for the journey. He proceeded to tell me that his partner had apprised him of my situation. That made me felt settled at this point, as I was now aware of communications between them. I knew for sure that my main urologist had my back, and the thought that he was going to make sure everything goes well, left me with a warm feeling.

The Male Sling

The male sling was introduced.

Up to this point my view and impression of the male sling continued to be fuzzy. My doctor then drew a simple but effective diagram to illustrate the system and how it actually works.

"After the procedure", he assured me, "you will go from zero to one pad per day".

My friends, I am a habitual coffee drinker. Whenever I do imbibe I enjoyed the quality of the beans and how it picks me up. The words from the doctor had the same *pick me up quality* and now I was ready to sign up.

In that short instance I had moved from the stage of a draftee to a willing volunteer. Zero to one pad a day! That I could live with for sure! Compared to what I was going through now, that would definitely be returning to normalcy.

The truth is men, we can survive prostate cancer and still lose our life. The life of a man. The life of being normal. The scourge of incontinence will put you in a worse-off state than a menstruating woman. She in a normal situation wears pads for only a few days of the month. There is also menopause where she gets a permanent break from pads. Compared to you, an incontinent man, who have to wear pads all the days of the month, and all the months of the year, and for the rest of your life to be buried with the thing. Now if that isn't a stinker, I do not know what is.

Millions of men today, who are healthy with the exception of incontinence, have arrived on the scene as a new breed of Homo Sapiens. They have burrowed themselves like ground hogs, back into some reclusive world. They only peek out when it is safe to do so. They operate in nocturnal fashion. They are introvertive and even scared. It is understandable then that these men have chosen to live less active lives, or forced to live less active lives, as another opinion might put it.

I could never, at this stage of my live become part of those statistics. The knowledge that I was gleaning, not only was it making me aware and wise but was providing me with buoyancy of a different kind. The kind that lifts my chin up and gives me hope. So, when the doctor gave me this first reconnaissance flyby, I was ready to drop the bomb on incontinence and all that it stands for. Indeed the mission was on, and I felt like a captain at the stern with the wind to my back.

As my understanding and knowledge goes, the male sling was introduced in 2006. Today it is used to treat patients with mild to moderate stress urinary incontinence resulting from radical prostatectomy.

This forms the basis of the treatment of which I was an immediate qualifier. The patient would have had to use more than one pad in 24 hours, over 40 years old, and has experienced stress urinary incontinence for at least 6 months.

The male sling is also an appropriate option for severely incontinent patients who are not candidates for the prosthetic option. Other conditions for treatment are that the patient must sign an agreement, give consent, willing and able to return for follow ups and evaluations. The patient must also be a good surgical candidate and the internal sphincter contractility must be confirmed by endoscopic views.

Unfortunately the procedure is not for everyone. People with bone deformation or other pathological conditions of the bone such as severe osteoporosis which would impair the securing of the bone screws, are in this group. If your immune system is compromised, and if there is any inflammation of the bone marrow, you would also be excluded. The procedure is also contraindicated in patients with urinary tract infections, upper or lower urinary tract obstruction or kidney failure or malfunction.

I have read testimonials from men who have gone through the procedure, who are and have been pleased with this procedure. The feedbacks attest to its safe, innovative and effective approach to immobilizing if not eradicating this problem of incontinence. Once it is affixed, it provides ventral compression of the urethra thus eliminating or greatly reducing urine leakage.

Another attractive feature of the male sling is that it involves minimally invasive surgery and one gets to go home the same day as mentioned before. The surgery is uncomplicated with high success rate and low complications. One can also elect for the application and use of only spinal anesthesia instead of general anesthesia. The procedure is also touted to allow for immediate outcome assessment and requires no patient activation or manipulation compared to the prosthetic treatment.

Fortunately for me, I fit these conditions perfectly. Frankly I was very relieved and delighted when my endoscopic view confirmed my contractility and my doctor made it known to me that I was *right for the procedure*.

By the turn of these events I had well cottoned up to this doctor and offered no resistance when he scheduled me right then and there, that same day, for surgery in two weeks time. Yes! There was nothing to think about, nothing to reconsider.

While there in his office I had read an article that said men who have this procedure experienced an improved sex life also. This was obviously an added bonus that I could store in my decision basket.

So with all these bonuses in tow, I told myself that I was securing my seat on this train. If it was midnight or morning it was not leaving me at this station of indecision. I was doused with a special feeling of euphoria. When they say "all on board" I knew I would not be left behind. Soon I hope to feel unfettered like a spy pigeon without the wire, and be able to fly again without the load and burden of urinary incontinence.

Chapter Nine

Monkey on my Back

For whatever the reasons were, I did not call my wife as soon as I got finished, as I was supposed to.

If I am honest with myself, maybe the reason was, that I had come upon a moment here.

I had walked out of that office cognizant of the fact that in a couple of weeks, I was going to be cut again. In spite of all the proposed benefits, the moment had now come to scald my back a bit. Something seemed to trail me from the doctor like a stalker that I could not see.

I had come down the elevator to the first floor walked through the lobby and exited right towards the parking garage where my vehicle was. My concern all the time was "What if..." What if I go through this and it does not work? What if I can't get 3 out of 3 and be perfect again? If these were normal thoughts, I do not know.
If under these circumstances your thoughts go places with you... I guess it is so...

However, before I could break out into a cold sweat, and before I was presented with a plaque of cowardice by some demon of indecision, before I drown in this sea of uncertainty, I began to swim again. There was a peak of an island in my view and soon I will be high and dry (physically and emotionally) so therefore I did not allow that negative gear to slow me down! I must find the strength now to swim for the shore of my life where I hope to begin to live normal again.

Many stories have been written about how the last lap is the hardest in a tough race and how some participants do not make it to the finish line.

Well I will be tarred and feathered if I allowed that to happen to me! So give way all you opposing and reactionary forces! Third base is in view my finish line is up ahead! This is PROSTATE CANCER AND ME…THE EXTRA MILE and by the help and strength of the one whose name alone is Jehovah; I am going to make it.

I had come to realize and to appreciate too, over the fifty something years of my life that most good things in life presented a fight in obtaining them. There are many ultra conservative forces that seem to protect the door of success like a flaming sword. And so be it, one has to put up a hard fight to go through that door of success

The fighting rules changed tremendously too when you have to fight against your very self to do what you must do to go through that door of success. One then probably has to pick his foot up and kick down that door to prevent him standing there like an abandoned package.

At this point I had arrived at a prideful recognition of self.
I had an appreciation that the process was complete now. I could lift myself off the shrink's couch for real and for good. There was the promise of a better life for me. In fact it was more like an assurance now, having met with the "sling man". As I alighted from the bowels of that dark parking garage and entered the beckoning world of light I experienced real optimism and hope.

The hole was sealed and plugged further by the thought of my two boys. They were two miniature versions of me and soon I could be running and playing with them in the park without going home too soon to change my wet behind. This had happened before where their objections and frowns on their little faces could not even prevent such an act on my part. It was hard to explain to them, a seven and a two year old that daddy has to go home and change his pad... Enough was enough! I had conquered prostate cancer as my insignificantly low PSA level readings showed. Now I must go on living life. I even managed a smile now instead of that constrained frown when I thought *this is my safari and I am going to whack and bag this monkey on my back.*

My Present To My Wife

After that introspective examination of self, I remembered that I should have called my wife. However, I still did not do that. I knew then that I wanted to see the girl, sit her down with me on the love seat and apprise her of this development. There were certain feelings of presenting her with a kind of special gift, and I wanted to make an occasion out of it.

I really felt that I had something special for her, particularly seeing that she did not know of this early date for the procedure.

So, all things considered, this was a gift. A special gift that I felt proud of. It was like finding the last ripe mango of the season on the mango tree, and it would be a travesty to eat it all by yourself.

This last mango, that you had to climb the tree to get.
It was hidden from everyone else by the tree leaves, and you by some act of God, was the only one to see it when the wind exposed its hiding spot.

Usually you would not share this mango with anyone but typically with a special someone, someone whom you love. In fact you would want to give it all to her. You would then wrap it up in newspaper after you have ingested a lungful of its aroma, and wait for the right moment to give it to her. This was my "last mango" of the season of prostate cancer and I hoped when I presented it to my wife that she would enjoy it, as how she would the succulence and prized taste of a last mango.

I had always prized myself as a tough son of the soil, but as I thought of what I will do, and the ends that I would go to make my wife happy some tears fell from my eyes and I couldn't understand why I was crying. I recognized again, though, that I really do love this woman.

The evening came. After my wife came home and the usual pleasantries were exchanged, naturally the question followed as appropriate as fire follows smoke. She asked "So, how did it go at the doctor's today?"

I proceeded to tell my wife everything. I told her how I couldn't even argue with the doctor about their tardiness in running the appointment scheme because he was a much nicer fellow than what the waiting room situation presented.

At this psychological moment, the moment of presenting her with "the mango", I said "my surgery is schedule in two weeks time".
She looked up at me with a pair of bright eyes and intoned "They didn't waste time did they?"

Her demeanor had also changed to such girlish anticipation as she changed sitting position and rested her head on my chest. She then looked into my eyes with a smile on her face that could melt the heart of an enraged bull, and maybe turn him into a puppy dog. My wife then said "Everything is going to be alright". She was enjoying this "last mango" for sure and my reaction was to have my face moved into a smile bigger than that of the full moon.

She then shifted smoothly into another gear. A gear of getting down to business. "Well" she said, "I'll have to take my two weeks vacation then, and it will run into the holidays for another week" looking up at me again she said, "Then I will be home with you for three weeks while you get well".

The smiley face returned to my face. I should have said "thank you" but instead hugged her closer to me. We sat there for a bit. We did not say anything. As she rubbed my arm wither her hand, something she always does when she is comfortable or contemplative, I could read her thoughts. Her thoughts of having me back as the man she knew.

The last time I came home from the doctor like this, from a consultation with the doctor and my wife meeting me home, was when I was diagnosed with prostate cancer. What a difference in mood that was! As I remembered this and returned to the heavy cloud of melancholy that associated the time, this moment gave me a thermal of hope, and anticipation. An involuntary swallow action in my throat affirmed to me that this was the right move. This "last mango" was indeed good! and the monkey on my back in this my personal safari, was as good as dead.

The Next Stage

The next stage of the game was the pre-admission test.
That is when thy check you out of course, and make sure that you are not going to have a heart attack, or bleed to death in the operation room or some other *out of the norm* development. I am a little cynical about these pre-admission tests and always thought what if they had to scoop my butt off the streets from some accident scene…would they be asking me those redundant questions and going through these tests? I am also curious of the situation where, if the insurance was not there as a lactating cow, what would these sessions be like or amount to!

Before I came to that though, I had to inform my mother, my mother-in-law and a few trusted and close friends, of my second fate with the knife. My mother was readily on board as she had always trusted me to make the right decisions. She however lamented over the fact that she might not be able to be with me this time, as she was with the first surgery.

My mother-in-law though, asked more questions. "Is it going to make you better?" she wanted to know. "Who is going to do it?". "Is it the same doctor?", were some of her queries.

I then explained what the deal was and emphasized the fact that I *got this*. She then resigned the interrogation and concluded in her usual thick Trinidadian accent, "Well boy, what ah go tell yuh? You have to do what you have to do".

So what if my mother-in-law is naturally more inquisitive than my mother? That is alright! I know she is a good person, as she has never taken her daughter to one side and question her, or, let her nose grow in our business. She has always wished me the best and supported me in my trials.

As the moon slept and the sun came to life, this was another particular morning.
They will fuss over me this morning.
This morning they will seek to give me clearance for the second landing on the operating table. Another sober milestone had crept upon me. The pre admission personnel were nice. In fact very nice, especially when my blood pressure readings came up as normal. Yes! The needle that I hate, the one they use to draw blood followed. (I was glad that I had insurance to pay for all of that). To complete the package of course, was all the medical questions that I had to answer.

At this point the displeasure of the moment was like a taste that you don't like at the back of the throat. I had in fact thought that this was going to be a simple procedure as was told to me. In my mind a simple procedure should be something like a snip, tuck and shut. It is easy to see then why my prevailing thought was *why all of this fuss*. One thing I can tell you is this, if they adopt this pre-admission procedure at airports the airways would be pronounced safer. (They probably could find insurance to pay for that too).

Once the pre-admission was completed I came upon another sense of great expectation. It reminded me of tracking preys in my native Jamaican bush as a young lad growing up. Assuredly when you see fresh signs, you know you are onto something and your heart beats faster, in expectation of the kill. Still you have to be calm as over excitement can ruin your day.

Everything before this had its own nebulous feelings. There were even uncertainties that the pre-admission tests created. One never knows what they will find in those tests, and depending on those findings, it can delay the surgery or prevent you from even having it. As the saying goes *you can be well until the doctor sees you.* So until the green light was given, unbeknownst to everyone else, I had unwillingly come upon this train-crossing of preventions and uncertainties again.

Prior to the surgery date I got a call from the hospital with the instructions of what not to do, and to do, before coming in on my surgery day. It was then that I was properly relieved realizing that they had not found anything wrong with me and that I could now move onward. I was now onward like a Christian soldier knowing that salvation was in reach. My salvation was the appreciation that I may never have to wear absorption pads in my underwear again!

Operation Morning And Deja Vu

The second operation morning in my life came around and in spite of the monkey on my back that I wanted to kill, and the last mango feelings of satisfaction, I knew I have been here before.

Sitting in the waiting room of this hospital, I have been here before, where you look out of one eye at everyone else as you wonder what they were in for. I have been here before where you almost say why me, where you wish you did not have to go through this, where you wish you could have turned the clock of time back to when you were healthy and young. Where you could run, jump and skip, and have fun. I have been here before in this room where you waited for your name to be called, and to be wheeled away. Where you hope everything goes well and that you will wake up relieved, if not better. I have been here before where the dread of the unknown unwittingly becomes your companion, but hope beckons you.

After a short while though, and after I was assimilated into the environs, I had now come to be imbued with this strange and unmitigated feelings of entitlement (because I have been here before).

I have been here before not in this very room per say. Most people, probably no one could have guessed that I had been operated on before, and as hope became my friend, and faith my comforter, I sat down and took my place among fellow sufferers.

I did not have to wait long in the waiting room. In fact they came and got me quick enough which I could appreciate. It did make me feel somewhat important as I left the other hapless souls wallowing in their various apprehensive feelings, and waiting for their summons to be wheeled away too. I gladly stepped up to the call of my name, like a recognized ninth grader student to be given a plaque for good citizenship.

At another time I would have thought they grabbed me quicker than the others because they might be thinking that I was going to run away. But I am too old for that type of cynicism now and only asked the lady if my wife could come along too. We then walked towards the intake room with the nurse in front, me in the middle, and my wife in the back. That formation I do believe was not by design, but if my wife was replaced by another person, all they would have to say was "dead man walking" to complete the ambiance of the fellow making that last walk before they snuff him out.

I am not a person to question the evidences of the good. To question the good as they did Jesus could be something sinister and evil. Those who questioned Jesus and the good that he did ended up killing him. I therefore became enlightened again at the prospect before me and the new life that awaits me, as we alighted upon this room, the intake room.

There was another gentleman in the room.

He could be in for the same thing, I thought, even though he appeared to have been around the block a few times more than me, and had visible signs of life's battles. It lends some comfort to know that I had a partner this time on the journey. Funny enough though we did not ask each other what we were in for, even after the mannerly greeting and some small talk. It must be some kind of etiquette that I am not aware of.

A few minutes rolled by and then marched in the *separatist attendant*. She could well have been a nurse, and I have no business speaking of her in harsh terms. However, my time had come when I had to be extricated from my wife, and had to tell her bye. I have been here before…and the sinking feeling that I got like a child been wrenched from its mother was no less severe.

I knew that my intake partner will not have those feelings. The poor fellow had seemed like a hardened honey farmer who had become immune to stings. What could also help him too was the fact that he had no wife with him but a son who spent all the time talking on his cell phone.

But my wife's eyes had seemed to say, "Be a good boy now and go with this nice nurse". She of course gave me a kiss, and I also took consolation from the thought that when I come back I will be a better person and a proper man to her. As she handed me over, she assured me that she will be there when I got back.

It was at this point that I realized that I was being taken before my partner. I wondered why of course and thought it was only fair for him to go before me. He was there before me and looked like he could use the head start. As I mentioned though I did not know what he was in for, and maybe he was waiting for an organ or something. I turned back to say to my leathery intake partner, "Hey buddy, take care you hear, and all the best to you". In a gravelly voice he wished me the same. I then sat on the wheel chair and just like that I was on my way to meet up with the other players in my second surgery.

It was not to be so fast though, as I was intercepted by another nurse sitting at her desk by a window overlooking the city. As I said, I have been here before. I started to have vivid reminders of the window overlooking the city and I-95 at the other hospital for the first time. I viewed this as a good omen. Strange, though, how some simple things can affect you so profoundly. The good omen was because at that window where I had spent some time, I was recuperating, and getting ready for home. Good omen indeed! Good omen. The last vestige of fear fell to the ground and was gone, finally.

There was a sudden resurgence of the old me and I commented to the nurse that she couldn't be claustrophobic at all in this room with this view. She agreed and mentioned how she liked it there. She asked me some more redundant questions, tagged me and told someone that I was ready.

Second Surgery And Going Home

I was not expecting any familiar face in the operating room. Not even the doctor's. It would have been nice if he was there to tell me everything was ok, but from my previous experience I pretty well knew that I was on my own now. What I was not expecting too, but which came as a sweet surprise, was the friendliness and jocularity of the nurses and the anesthesiologist. The anesthesiologist even told me that the male nurse who put the drip receptacle in my arm was a crazy man. I told him to leave the fellow alone because he was alright with me. Realizing that he had Berlin wall to hide behind, the fellow hurled back, "Yeah! Leave me alone!" And here I am in typical fashion defending the underdog, even when immobilized and on my back!

Common prudence should have had me saying something like "Yeah he looks crazy to me", siding with the one who had my life in his hands. So for all intents and purposes, this horse had shot through the gate and I couldn't catch him even if I wanted to. The anesthesiologist had the last laugh though when he gave me the mask and turn my lights out.

I woke up from the surgery with the predicted uncomfortableness. I waited for the pains. I even call myself bracing for the pains. My doctor came to tell me that the procedure went very well and I will be going home in a few more hours. At first I did not recognize him. His nomenclature as the sling man had properly eluded me at this moment. It was not until he talked with the usual militaristic opulence that it clicked that this was the sling man. Who could have blamed me! I had never seen him covered in all those white stuff before, and devoid of his hard sole boots!

I wanted him to linger a bit so that I could ask some question (at least that was what my mind told me) but in a flash he was gone like Flash Gordon of comic book fame. Immediately after his disappearance, the angel of hope entered.

My tall, lanky, and beautiful wife.

I thought that by now the pains would have come but it was only a nauseous feeling and the stiffness of my hip joints that I was aware of. In my previous operation of the prostatectomy, by now I would be hollering like a pig with a kitchen knife stabbed in his behind. So I find it strange indeed that there were no severe pains accompanying this experience.

It was not without difficulty however, that I got onto the wheelchair after a while, with my discharged papers in tow and secured by my wife.

I was on my way home. A beautiful feeling indeed.
I had to take a seat on a hostile iron bench at the valet stand, while we wait for the vehicle. That by itself was not a nice experience. By now I was feeling a significant degree of discomfort and wished I was lying down instead of sitting, and on this cold, hard, iron bench. It was with difficulty that I got into the vehicle and understandably so, given the circumstances of my day.

My wife took me home like a lioness moving her cub to a safer den. She obviously had learned from the previous experience and was duly cautious about swerving and very watchful for potholes. As she maneuvered this bigger vehicle into the driveway of our house it was a job well done.

As I walked into our house that evening, I was immersed with the realization that now I did have the option to live again. That I did take the step not to be overreached by my depressing state of incontinence. I had actually fought back and was on my way to the podium to accept and claim my prize. There was a tremendous feeling of a fundamental accomplishment. This feeling gave me such an updraft and positivity that totally erased any of my previous doubts. My empowerment had returned and I felt that I was not sick anymore. Yes, I even felt that I had a right to be happy.

Home Again

Suffice it to say it was a good feeling to be home. This is where the journey could take on either an incline or a decline. I was not experiencing any factor that could have contributed to a decline. The nauseous feelings had long gone and I was mentally ready to climb back into the saddle. With no pains at all, I was looking forward to a speedy recovery. In fact I could lay at the front of my lair like a contended predator sensing the various offers of spring. What a big difference it was compared to when I had to retreat to the back of my lair in the first surgery, licking the wounds of recovery.

No more of that dark world of suffering and misery for me. It was over. I did have time to contemplate the most difficult evening of that period though, and that was when I left the hospital.

I had made it out of the vehicle gingerly and slowly. I probably looked like a constipated bull dog with my face contorted and walking wide. There was a cut beneath me that could be expressed colloquially as in my undercarriage, which rendered me like a turkey prepared for stuffing.

There were pains in my hip joints from the position that I was straddled in, to get to my undercarriage. As I reminisce about this I could appreciate the gruesome sight as they hooked me up and split me from my scrotal bag to my anus ring. That explains the discomfort in my hip joints and why I had to stay wide. Coupled with that fact too, was the hospital dressing on my undercarriage, which encouraged me to keep my legs from getting close.

I will take that any day as I was not feeling anything close to what I had felt in the first surgery.

I wouldn't say I felt like clicking my heels, in a jump of ecstasy and elation, as to be operated on is no joke under most circumstances.

Whether it is invasive or non-invasive your body will still complain and tell you it does not like to be cut. Correctly so too as nothing can compensate for the normal and original you. My psychological feeling of well being , however continued to present a warmth of a rising sun and I felt that my days of urinary incontinence were all boxed up, and ready to be launched off like space junk, into an unreachable orbit.

My discharging instructions from the hospital were clear and precise. I did not know that, partly because I did not read them and partly because I have a hawk for a wife, who swooped down and took them from the discharger's hand. Later on I will learn that she would use them against me like how a lawyer uses a contract.

I remembered the doctor saying that I should abstain from sex for a period of six weeks and I should not lift anything greater than ten pounds. In consultation with him before the surgery, I did recall the emphasis he had placed on me taking it easy after the surgery to assist in the healing of the scar tissue, and enhancing the ventral compression of the urethra. In lay terms the scar tightening around the urethra is central in correcting that big hole through which the urine flow uncontrollably. The contractibility of the muscles would then return giving me control once again. So "take it easy" he had cautioned.

The doctor also said "If the tightening comes loose and heals back with the hole the surgery from all angle would have been a failure". And so all of that I got. No sex! No lifting! And take it easy! Nowhere in that did it say that I should go home and become a vegetable, as my hen-hawk wife wanted me to be.

My wife had hawkeyed other instructions for my recovery from the discharge papers, that I got bellowed to me whenever I was guilty of even the smallest infraction. Honestly, some of those rules I thought she had made up until I had a chance to read them one day. I could then see why she was scalding my hide with reproof and admonition.

After those instructions and information bit into my consciousness, a moment with myself at this point went like this. *Goodness gracious me! This was a minor procedure. All those instructions about don't stretch, don't climb up into a vehicle. Maybe they should have said don't speak to a stranger either, then I would have gotten it more quickly and more complete.* For all intents and purposes the depth of my simple procedure had all but eluded me.

Before this conscious moment in time, I could not appreciate my wife's vested interest in my recovery and the success of my surgery. Remember she was very disenchanted about all that watery sex and flooded bed that we used to have. My desire to keep some kind of mobility going and to not keep company with a vegetative state, invariably clashed with her desire, and would result in tumbling balls of conflicts.

For the time that she was home with me, if I was ever caught downstairs I would get a piece of tongue lashing and admonition that made me felt like the puppy that peed on the carpet.
After a while, any gainful entrance to the kitchen and downstairs had to be artfully contrived or ingeniously planned. The coast had to be completely clear.

It meant then that she couldn't be anywhere in the house or its environs, and only then could I go downstairs for a drink of water or a biscuit with some cheese. *"Stealth"* indeed, became my modus operandi! Not to mention hiding the evidences of my incriminations to make such mission a successful one! Failure to have all those conditions working in sync would always have me taking from her :
"The doctor says...", "Your discharge instructions say..." , and "I say...". She would shove all that down my throat like some unsavory bush medicine my grandmother used to make me take.

The tumbling balls of conflicts would only end, when I throw in the white towel, and she would walk away with her tail in the air, like a muskrat matriarch, and I would be left in the state of the puppy that peed on the carpet, and got caught by his owner. She would always win. After my dismal defeat if I did not voluntarily depart upstairs and back into bed, she would stretch her 5 feet 10 inches frame over me and with her pointing finger like a bayonet, marched me back upstairs.

As I got better and she softened on me a bit, I was only allowed downstairs after she was properly apprised of my intentions.

She would then afford and supply visual and physical supervision to ensure my safe landing. What a woman! It is no wonder that I love her so…

These scenes reminded me of growing up when visiting a friend with a bad dog in his yard, you have to call out before you get close, and probably climb a tree so the dog wouldn't get you. He would then have to tie up the dog and you can go visit. Otherwise, entering such a friend's yard could result in that dog knowing what you taste like. Albeit hen hawk or bad dog, this woman loves me and I love her too, and I do appreciate the attention she gave me. I would venture to say that if a fly had perched on me she would have killed it!

Oh yes! She worked that beat alright. Not even the boys were exempted. Oftentimes their crimes of jumping up and down on the bed with me on it, earned them severe Trinidadian-type tongue lashings and marching orders to their room with this reminder sealing their fate "your father is sick!"

My wife's interest in me and this stage of recovery was seeded in the fact that I had told her, and showed her, that there was no leakage.

There was absolutely no urine flow.

This called for a celebration of some sorts and I later did that with a glass of red and enjoyed its mellow taste for the first of a long time.

To my delight the red stayed in me and did not respond to the pulls of gravity as it had done in the past almost two years. Michael Jackson had said "This is it" for his optimum tour. On that same page I was asking,

"Could this be it?"

"Did I really have one foot back in the stirrup, and was getting ready to mount back in the saddle?"

Arguably I was experiencing a deep sense of anticipation. I did not want to put this news on the lighthouse top as yet though as I knew this was only the morning after. I will wait and see. I was now sitting up at the entrance to my lair, ready to be a force to be reckoned with once again! Ready to be redeployed into the world of moustache muscle!

Of course the sitting down, getting up, lying down standing up "Simon Says" game continued for about a week or so. Gradually though, my mobility improved and so I could wade into the deeper waters of the living. Right quickly I was able to make tea and fry an egg. With two slices of whole wheat bread in the mix, that was breakfast. I even used the sitting-down/standing-up method to cook dinner one evening and surprised my wife when she got home. By the end of the 6th week I felt wind in my sail again. I couldn't slay a dragon yet though but was ready to tease him from afar. So gradually and rather quickly too, I was able to stand up longer and take short gingerly walks.

My follow up check with the doctor came.
Sitting down in his office that morning he said to me "Well Lloyd, how are you doing?"
"Doc!" I answered excitedly, "I do not know what you did, but I have not leaked since the morning of the surgery."

My doctor, the man that he is and all, showed an emotion that was devoid of everything doctorial, but resorted to such admirable level of empathy, when he got up from his chair, walked around the table, stooped over me and gave me a hug. He then said "I am happy for you man".

It was a blessed and glorious day when I chose this group of doctors. I knew it then from the first surgery but confirmed it now and once again. I couldn't find the right words to express my gratitude to him but found myself expressing these inadequate words "Thank you Doc".

His affirmative hug, his assurance, his squeeze had indicated to me that we had scored the goal.

The rubble of incontinence that buried me for almost 2 years was finally lifted off me by this man, this doctor, and all I could say was thank you. The real sense of gratitude was totally snuffed by those terse words. My only relief from the inability to really express to him how I felt was when I realize that there were no words or expression in the English language to properly convey my sentiments.

We continued to have light conversations about the prescribed course of my recovery. He reiterated what I should or should not do. Those instructions include of course no sexual activity for 6 weeks. Of course feeling the little wind in my sail I said to him, "Doc, what am I to do with this young wife?" I always like to have the doctors' wording on such delicate matter so that I can quote them to her. "Put her on a slow cooker for now", he said.

That evening I decided to give her the warning before the rain cloud sets. Before her emotions break the levees and rushed her towards me. It was only fair to have her warned so that she will continue her firm perch on that ledge, before jumping off and there is no water in the pool.

"The doctor said I should put you on a slow cooker for now. You will leave me alone until I healed up right!" I told her. All that she did was to giggle and said "I know. Remember I read the discharge papers". It was then I realized that she had already put herself on a slow cooker.

It is now three months since I had the male sling placed inside me. Aside from the occasional tightness in the mornings, which is loosened up once I get on the move, everything continued to be normal.

I feel I am finally set now for the course of the rest of my life, unimpeded by incontinence. It is difficult to describe the feelings of euphoria that I get at times from the regained ability to control my urine flow.

A lot of men today live normal and healthy lives. Mine was such too until I was unceremoniously jettisoned by prostate cancer. As a healthy man, I did not take the ability or inability to control my urine flow to be of nay importance or significance. By all means what healthy men do is eat, drink, sleep, work, maybe exercise. We take these functions of our body for granted. But an old Jamaican saying goes like this *cow never knows the use of its tail until it is chopped off*. Likewise for me, I never knew how important it was to me to control my urine until I lost it.

This experience made me reflect on the fact that I am wonderfully made! This has enabled me not to take even the simplest things for granted, especially where my health is concerned.
Three months after the surgery I continued the happy life of not wearing absorption pads and all the other demerits associated with that. I do not have to worry anymore about that thing of incontinence and found that I am not depressed by feelings of inadequacies.

Recently I returned to one of the scenes of my personal and private disgrace. It was the round–robin trip to a friend's house outside the city. Our last visit to this place had me performing on a stage of make belief. I made belief that the wine that I drank was not running through me like a waterfall. That my pants were not wet, and that I was enjoying myself. On this occasion though, I boasted at the dinner table that I was not peeing on myself. The wine that I was drinking actually stayed in me… and gave me a soothing, and comfortable buzz.

Chapter Ten

Conclusion

Prostate Cancer...and You?

Prostate Cancer and Me is a story I felt compelled to tell, to encourage every male to take this matter seriously. I realize from my own circle of contemporaries that we are still ignorant and very much behind the bush where this disease is concerned. The bush is burning, but too many of us are still wearing sandals.

They used to say that prostate cancer is an old man's disease. We now know that is not so. More younger men than ever before are developing it. So let us bury that notion, and realize instead the accepted facts that it is a cumulative disease, in some cases hereditary, and that life- style choices or actions starting as early as boyhood can be part of the picture.

Some statistics say that one in three men will have some prostate issue, from enlargement to cancer. And if you ask your doctor he will tell you that fifty percent of men over age fifty will have the disease. These statistics are even more staggering for black men—so much so, that in some circles it is dubbed "the black man's disease."

In Great Britain when something wise and commendable is achieved or carried out, the appreciative observer exclaims, "Brilliant!" I think the opposite of "brilliant" is "foolish or stupid." As a man, I decided with the help of my wife to be brilliant and live, and not to be stupid and die. The beginning of being brilliant (and living) is to go for regular checkups with your doctor. And if your doctor wants you to have further tests under the care of a specialist, go for the further tests.

An allegedly wise person I know told me that he couldn't go through another biopsy after experiencing the first one. What might have happened to me if I had taken that course! For crying out loud! There are many men in the world like my allegedly wise friend. Some have not even checked to see the status of their PSA level, which can be discerned through a simple blood test . Here's another point along those lines: According to my doctor, 20% of men polled said they would never have had the cancer surgery operation had they known the aftermath—the pain and discomforts that had to be endured for a while. This is not being brilliant and living; this is being stupid and risking dying.

There should be only one ostrich, and that is the bird. There should be no ostrich-men, men who are aware of this disease, but nevertheless stick their heads in the proverbial sand and do nothing about it. We should be men who rise to the fore in the name of good health for the sake of our loved ones, and for the sake of other men who can follow our lead and example. Remember that it took many trials before man could be landed on the moon, and say, "One small step for man, one giant leap for man-kind." Then Houston could later say, "Mission accomplished." We should not leave our PSA level status in the wings, but throw this machismo stuff out the window, continue to take that one small step every year to the doctor to be tested, and contribute to making that giant leap for all men.

Some Final Thoughts

Over the months I've described in this book, I learned a lot about the prostate gland and prostate cancer. Some things I learned from speaking with doctors and other professionals, and some I learned on my own, through experiences and research. So I feel that I am in a good position to add some further thoughts and advice on the matter. Such falls into two categories: first, steps you can take right now to help keep your prostate gland healthy, and second, what you should know and what you can do if you are beginning treatment for prostate cancer.

What To Do To Decrease the Risk

The old adage that prevention is better than the cure, in my opinion, should be strongly heeded regarding prostate cancer. As of now, the prevention piece has been as elusive as Bigfoot. However, while there are no clear-cut preventative procedures to take, it is widely agreed that actions in several areas can be tremendously helpful in staving off the disease. You don't have to wait until your doctor says, "Your PSA level is high," to minimize your chances of ever hearing that report in the first place. These actions are the following:

Maintain a proper diet.
In the course of my journey through the medical world, I learned that the prostate is one of the most sensitive glands in the male body. It is sensitive to the steroids and hormones often used to produce foods made of beef, pork, and chicken. Therefore, it would seem to be wise not to purchase these foods in a mindless fashion, grabbing whatever comes to hand, but to check to see what the farmer or producer uses in raising their animals or in growing vegetable crops. Suffice it to say that a man shouldn't be eating anything that is not produced or grown naturally or organically.
A few friends of mine actually have decided to purchase only meat that they can first see alive. They interview the farmer about what he feeds his animals or what type fertilizer he uses on his plants, sometimes asking to see evidence. After all, as one of them told me, "You are what you eat." He is so right!
I know that my diet as an adult had seriously deviated from my childhood diet of fruits, vegetables, beans, fish, and meat

that we either hunted or grew ourselves, usually without the artificial fertilizers that the modern world now uses. For too long, my diet had since those days taken a turn to the bonanza of available cheap meats and other food products available through mass production with the help of steroids, hormones, fertilizers, insecticides, and more.

Exercise regularly.
Also as an adult, I was going to the gym to bulk up, as I had always wanted to be a force to be reckoned with, and I did little or no jogging after leaving my teenage stage. We now know that "bulking up" exercises do not seem to help the prostate, while running or jogging with the abdominal and pelvic muscles in play is strongly recommended to help keep the prostate in ticking fashion.

So another wise step is adding some aerobic exercise to a gym routine that maybe has focused on weight training and the like.

Have regular sex.
When we were boys, and particularly when entering puberty, we passed through a period that is commonly recognized by wet dreams, when a dream of having sex leads to ejaculation. Most men will tell you that as a young boy this happened to them regularly. It has been believed that wet dreams are one way the prostate rids itself of built-up sperm and seminal fluids. And indeed, modern research indicates that ejaculation may reduce the risk of cancer by flushing out chemicals that enter the gland through the blood.

Once you start to wet the sheets with semen, your prostate gland has come into bloom. This is one sure sign that your prostate is now saying, "Start paying attention to me or I later on might kill you!" The question then is, why shouldn't men continue with this regular flushing of the prostate gland?

It was emphasized to me by an alternative health specialist that
not emptying the prostate regularly through sex—and the anger
associated with not having sex—is indeed a loaded gun for
prostate cancer.

In reflecting on my past, I drew connections to my own history.
I was probably one of the only boys growing up on the
Caribbean island of Jamaica who did not have a girlfriend. At
times this was embarrassing, as I couldn't contribute to the tales
of conquest and male prowess that were told by other boys.
When I grew up and went to college, I had another sex drought
of three years. Getting married to my first wife didn't help either,
as that experience was like walking through the desert with only
the occasional oasis on the way—maybe once a month.

I cannot blame anyone but myself for having an un-flushed
prostate for long periods of time. Had I known of the serious
health consequences it could bring, I am quite sure I could have
and would have done something about it.

Put all this together—diet, exercise, sexual activity—and the recipe for
prostate cancer could be realized as written for me. And boy, was
I eating from its table!

Given the fact that no male in my family line, going back three
generations, had ever been diagnosed with prostate cancer or died from
the disease...given the fact that their lifestyles were ones of physicality
and a diet of home-grown, healthfully produced foods...and given the
fact, yes, of their regular prostate flushing, as evidenced by the many
children they left behind, all this to me presented a con- trolled
experiment in which the results were obvious.
At my expense, certain factors in this experiment of my life cannot and
should not be overlooked or underestimated. It is absolutely
imperative to turn attention to that delicate but vital part of us that we

call the prostate gland. Consider this a plaintive wail from some- one who has been there and done that for you to take heed.

Now, suppose you have learned at your checkup that your PSA level is high, and further tests and examinations have revealed the presence of cancer. You will surely receive informed advice from your doctor about the options available to you. See a second doctor or a third, if that is necessary to help you reach a clear decision on how to proceed.

In most cases, surgery is likely to be recommended. What then?

What to Do If You Have Prostate Cancer

I have written my story here in detail, to "tell it like it is." Or to tell it in a way that you might not hear from your doctor, no matter how skilled and excellent a physician he or she is, or from the nurses and other medical staff involved in your care. This is not because they are unfeeling or unsympathetic, but because their job, first and foremost, is to detect the disease and to use all the modern methods at their disposal to eradicate it. Their focus is not primarily on the side effects, mental and physical.

What I have described in the pages you have just read is the inside story, the story of what you may experience in your body and in your mind as you undergo treatment. The better prepared you are ahead of time with clear information about what to expect, the better equipped you will be to take measures that will help you enormously, both in the immediate aftermath of surgery and on the longer road ahead to restored health, strength, and vigor.

So let me in these final pages pull together the lessons I learned:

(1) Ask questions of your medical team.

Do not hesitate to request all the information you need. Too often, we think we shouldn't "bother" these experts with our concerns.

(2) If you are in pain, ask for medication.
And if the medication prescribed isn't doing the job, ask for something more powerful. Don't be a hero, gritting your teeth through great pain because that seems the "manly" thing to do.

(3) After surgery, while still in the hospital, try to start walking as soon as you can.

Even if you have to push yourself a little and even if your walking is mostly a shuffle. Keep moving, because moving helps your circulation and breathing, and promotes healing.

(4) Be prepared to experience some negative psychological effects of spending perhaps several days in the hospital. It can be sad and even depressing to live in an environment of illness. Try to maintain positive spirits and try, too, to empathize with those who are going through their own difficult time.

(5) Prostate cancer surgery and its aftermath is a family affair!

Yes, you are the main actor in this drama, but your wife, mother, children, whatever loved ones are close to you are dealing with their own reactions, concerns, and fears. Try to help them, and let them help you.

(6) If a loss of sexual desire or potency is extremely disheartening and important to you and/or your wife, talk to your doctor about it.
Do not be embarrassed about these issues and about requesting help.
(7) If urinary incontinence is disheartening and the need to wear absorbency pads is making you feel like a baby, make the best of it. It won't last forever. Change the pads often. Pick up some

cornstarch powder to make that area feel less irritated.

(8) Prepare for a relatively long healing time.
You will be advised to refrain from any heavy lifting or manual labor for a while. But you may also find yourself trying to return to your usual routines, only to feel suddenly and unnaturally fatigued and not quite up to things as normal. This is par for the course. Give yourself time.

(9) Look for a support team.
Even if you are someone who has never been inclined to gather in talk groups, there can be great comfort in sharing your story with others who have been on the same journey, in hearing their stories, and in realizing you are not alone.

(10) Be thankful for your life.

Men of the world, men of the nations, men of tribes and tongues, men mostly young or not so old, whether you can kill a lion or only swat a fly: Hear ye! Hear ye! Hear ye! Hear this as the last call before the black curtain falls! This story I must tell, so that it rings a bell, so that it sends a warning for you to heed, in haste and speed.

There could be a bullet inside you loaded in an air trigger gun, depending on how you act or how you fail to act. Once that bullet is fired, you cannot stop it nor can you outrun it.

It is not that proboscis between your legs that makes you a man. It is not the size of it, the name you call it, or your seeming prowess. It is that little gland called the prostate. Men! Say hello to your little friend!

Not paying attention to that little gland, your little friend, disrespecting the pivotal role it plays in your life, can cut you down and cause you to fall like another timber in the forest.

Be scared!

And then be smart!

Man to man, prostate cancer and me does not have to be prostate cancer and you.

ABOUT THE AUTHOR

Lloyd Martin is a native of Jamaica, who was born in Mason Hall district in the parish of St. Mary. He had a successful career in teaching in his native country, where his particular impact was made at Tivoli Gardens High 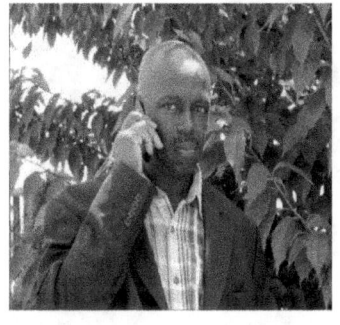 School as a young teacher from Excelsior Community College. He continued his work and education at the University of the West Indies where he was certified in Marketing and Public Relations.

Upon Lloyd's arrival in the USA in 1988, he made a conscious, yet long thought out decision to leave his beloved profession of teaching and pursued a path in financial services. Working through the ranks he moved from sales rep with Metropolitan Life to area manager with Surety Life. Continuing in the financial service field, he later became a mortgage broker specializing in residential and commercial mortgages.

With the advent of Prostate Cancer, Lloyd Martin had to take the full count on one knee. However he is back again in the saddle, spurned on by the spirit of life and entrepreneurism. He continues to be an encouraging source to his contemporaries through the talks and speeches he gives.

Lloyd Martin is also a registered advocate for the fight against cancer with the American Cancer Society. He has also appeared as guest speaker on radio talk shows on America's east and west coast.